HEART HEALTHY
COOKBOOK FOR BEGINNERS

1500 Days of Delicious and Easy Recipes

to Lower Your Blood Pressure and Cholesterol Level

MELISSA WESTWOOD

TABLE OF CONTENTS

Introduction 9

What to Eat and What Not to Eat 9

BREAKFAST RECIPES 11

Spinach Omelet 12

Roasted Vegetable and Egg Skillet 12

Lentil Asparagus Omelet 13

Eggs in an Avocado 14

Shrimp Salad with Avocado 14

Peanut Butter Banana Oatmeal 15

Creamy Millet Porridge with Berries 15

Apricot Granola with Fresh Fruit 16

Smashed Peas, Avocado, and Egg Toast 17

Coconut Milk Pudding 17

Apple Cinnamon Quinoa Breakfast Bowl 18

Spinach & Egg Scramble with Raspberries 19

Carrot Baked Oatmeal 19

Bagel Avocado Toast 20

Southwestern Waffle 21

Pineapple-Grapefruit Detox Smoothie 21

Pistachio & Peach Toast 22

Overnight Matcha Oats with Berries 23

Strawberry Peach Smoothie 23

Breakfast Parfait 24

Almond Butter & Roasted Grape Toast 24

Healthy Bread Pudding 25

Muesli with Raspberries 25

Cannellini Bean & Herbed Ricotta Toast 26

Egg Tartine 27

Candied Apples 27

Tofu Scramble 28

Raspberry Mousse 29

Summer Berry Parfait with Yogurt 29

LUNCH RECIPES 31

Chicken and Pesto Sourdough Sandwich 32

Turkey and Spinach Rice Bowl 32

Two-Mushroom Barley Soup 33

Hearty White Bean and Kale Soup 33

Chicken and Rice Stew 34

Fried Chicken Bowl 35

Baked Mustard-Lime Chicken 35

Easy Keto Korean Beef with Cauli Rice 36

Chicken with Mushroom Sauce 37

Asian Chicken Lettuce Wraps 38

Pan-Seared Pork and Fried Tomato Salad 38

Bourbon Steak 39

Fish Chowder Sheet Pan Bake 40

Maple Salmon 41

Hawaiian Chop Steaks 41

Shrimp Capellini 42

Chopped Power Salad with Chicken 43

Honey Walnut Chicken 44

Black Bean Risotto.. 45

Cilantro-Lime Chicken and Avocado Salsa................................. 46

Green Beans and Mushrooms Spaghetti...................................... 47

Balsamic Rosemary Chicken 48

Turkey Sandwich 49

Salmon and Summer Squash in Parchment 49

Rainbow Trout Baked in Foil... 50

Sesame-Crusted Tuna Steaks 51

Salmon and Scallop Skewers.. 52

Shrimp Scampi with Zoodles 53

Lemon Garlic Mackerel... 54

Broiled Tuna Steaks with Lime.. 55

Oven-Roasted Salmon Fillets... 56

Moroccan Spiced Chicken with Onions....................................... 56

Spaghetti Squash and Chickpea Sauté.. 57

Grilled Chicken Breasts with Plum Salsa................................... 59

Pesto Pasta 59

Chicken Kebabs Mexicana.. 60

Chicken Cutlets with Pineapple Rice 61

DINNER RECIPES 63

Oven-Roasted Salmon with Vinaigrette 64

Portobello Mushrooms with Mozzarella 64

Chicken Kebabs 65

Indian Spiced Cauliflower Fried Rice 66

Tofu Vegetable Stir-Fry 67

Pocket Eggs with Sesame Sauce 68

Lentil Walnut Burgers 69

Zucchini "Spaghetti" with Almond Pesto 70

Farro with Sun-Dried Tomatoes 71

One-Skillet Quinoa and Vegetables 72

Tarragon Sweet Potato and Egg Skillet 73

Black-Eyed Pea Collard Wraps with Sauce 74

Braised Cauliflower and Squash Penne 75

Mushroom Frittata 76

Egg, Carrot, and Kale Salad Bowl 77

Grilled Squash Garlic Bread 78

Turkish-Style Minted Chickpea Salad 79

Thai Chicken Salad 80

Cauliflower Fried Rice 81

Salmon with Creamy Feta Cucumbers 82

Chicken Salad with Pistachios 83

Tilapia with Tomatoes and Pepper Relish 84

Simple Tomato Basil Soup 85

Creamy Chicken and Chickpea Salad 86

Seared Tilapia with Spiralized Zucchini 86

Broccoli and Gold Potato Soup 87

Braised Lentils and Vegetables 88

Acorn Squash Stuffed with White Beans 89

Cheesy Artichoke Toasts 90

Spring Minestrone Soup 91

Lemon-Thyme Chicken 92

Roasted Garlic and Tomato Lentil Salad 93

Grilled Chicken and Cherry Salad 94

Creamy Asparagus Pea Soup 95

Pork Fried Rice 96

Chicken Satay 97

Easy Fried Eggplant 98

Simple Lemon-Herb Chicken 99

Rustic Vegetable and Bean Soup 99

Easy Chorizo Street Tacos 100

Moroccan Spiced Red Lentils Stew 101

Garlic Ranch Chicken 102

Flounder Tacos with Cabbage Slaw 103

Easy Baked Tilapia 104

Tuna Fish Pea Salad 104

Loaded Sweet Potatoes 105

Creamy Quinoa, Lentils, and Vegetables 106

Shrimp and Rice Noodle Salad 108

Roasted New Red Potatoes 110

Potato Dumplings 110

Marinated Carrot Salad 111

Tofu Salad 112

Tomato Cucumber Salad 113

Quinoa Spinach Power Salad 113

Salad of Kale, Avocado, and Carrots 114

Fruit Punch Salad 115

Avocado and Eggs Salad 116

Gingered Beef and Broccoli Salad Bowl 117

Spinach, Pears, and Cranberries Salad 118

Zucchini Patties 118

Sweet and Spicy Tofu Salad with Carrot 119

Marinated Cucumber & Tomato Salad 120

Wilted Spinach and Tilapia Salad 121

30-DAY MEAL PLAN 122

Introduction

A healthy diet is an essential part of living a healthy life. Eating a diet that is good for your heart can lower your risk of heart disease and other health problems like high blood pressure and diabetes.

A heart-healthy diet has many different parts, but some of the most important things to focus on are eating a lot of fruits and vegetables, cutting back on saturated and trans fats, and choosing lean sources of protein.

What to Eat and What Not to Eat

We are what we eat, which is no mystery. Food has a direct impact on both our physical and emotional health. That's why it's important to consider what we put in our bodies. There are some foods that are widely thought to be healthier than others, even if there are no hard-and-fast rules on what to eat and what to avoid.

A vital food for our bodies is protein. It produces enzymes and hormones, aids in tissue growth and repair, and gives our DNA structure. Meat, poultry, fish, eggs, dairy products, beans, nuts, and seeds are all the best sources of protein.

It's critical to select protein-rich foods that are low in cholesterol and saturated fat. Good options include lean meats, skinless chicken, fish, tofu, lentils, and low-fat or fat-free dairy products.

It's crucial to keep in mind that we need to restrict our intake of some protein sources. Red and processed meats like bacon and sausage contain a lot of cholesterol and saturated fat and should only be consumed in moderation.

One nutrient that is frequently forgotten when it comes to eating for health is fiber. Everyone should strive to get roughly 25 g of fiber every day because it is an essential component of a balanced diet.

Soluble and insoluble fibers are both available. When soluble fiber dissolves in water, a gel-like substance is produced that can aid in slowing down digestion and keeping you fuller for longer. Insoluble fiber helps to add weight to your stool, which can aid with bowel regularity because it does not dissolve in water.

Fruits, vegetables, legumes, whole grains, nuts, and legume products are just a few examples of foods that contain fiber. Black beans, lentils, broccoli, Brussels sprouts, oats, chia seeds, and flaxseeds are a few examples of foods high in fiber. By simply substituting some refined carbs in your diet, you may easily add extra fiber to it.

Consuming enough fiber is essential for overall health and wellbeing. Fiber intake has been demonstrated to reduce the risk of obesity, type 2 diabetes, heart disease, and stroke. Additionally, fiber can help decrease cholesterol and maintain healthy blood sugar levels. So, bear it in mind the next time you prepare a meal or a snack.

It's best to stay as far away from added sugar as you can. Limiting sweetened foods and beverages like candy, cake, and soda is necessary to achieve this. Instead, choose naturally sweet meals like fruits and vegetables. If you do consume items with added sugar, make sure to counterbalance them with healthier foods to avoid overdosing on your body.

BREAKFAST

RECIPES

Spinach Omelet

Preparation time: 10 minutes   Cooking time: 5 minutes

Ingredients:

- 2 slices of whole grain bread
- 1/2 of avocado (100g)
- 2 oz low-sodium smoked salmon (56g)
- salt and pepper to taste.
- lemon juice (optional)

Directions:

1. Toast the bread slices until they are crisp.
2. Remove the pit from the avocado, cut it in half, and scoop the flesh into a small bowl. Mask it with a fork until smooth.
3. Spread the mashed avocado evenly on the bread.
4. Top with low-sodium smoked salmon.
5. Optionally, add a few drops of lemon juice on top.

Nutrition: Calories: 108; Fat: 8.75g; Carbs: 0.6g; Protein: 6.35g

Roasted Vegetable and Egg Skillet

Preparation time: 10 minutes   Cooking time: 7 minutes

Ingredients:

- 1/2 tbsp olive oil (7ml)
- 1½ cups mixed vegetables (broccoli, carrots, bell pepper, spinach) (150g)
- 1/2 tbsp garlic powder or fresh minced garlic
- Salt and pepper to taste
- 2 eggs (organic or omega-3 enriched)
- 2 tbsp fresh parsley or cilantro (8g)

Directions:

1. Turn on the grill. Heat the olive oil in a medium baking dish or broiler-safe pan.

2. Add the garlic powder and veggies. Add salt and pepper, then lightly toss to coat.

3. After about 2 minutes, stir the skillet and cook it for an additional 2 minutes under the broiler on the center oven shelf.

4. Bring the pan out of the oven, top with eggs, and put it back under the broiler.

5. Broil until cooked to your liking: for over easy eggs, about 2 to 3 minutes.

6. Watch closely as the eggs will cook quickly.

7. Divide the vegetable and egg mixture between two serving plates, top with the fresh cilantro, and serve immediately.

Nutrition: Calories: 121; Fat: 8.5g; Carbs: 7g; Protein: 7g

Lentil Asparagus Omelet

Preparation time: 15 minutes   Cooking time: 20 minutes

Ingredients:

- 2 eggs, whisked
- 1/2 tbsp dried thyme
- 2 tbsp sliced onion
- 1/2 cup sliced asparagus (125g)

- 1/4 cup rinsed and drained lentils (50g)
- 1/4 sliced grape tomatoes (37g)
- 4 thin avocado slices (30g)

Directions:

1. Whisk together eggs and thyme in a bowl and set aside.

2. Preheat a nonstick skillet over medium heat.

3. Sauté onion and asparagus for 2-3 minutes.

4. Add legumes and cook for another 2 minutes.

5. Reduce heat to keep the mixture warm.

6. In another pan over medium heat, add half of the egg mixture. Cook for 2-3 minutes.

7. Transfer the omelet to a plate.

8. Repeat with the remaining ingredients for the second omelet.

9. Garnish with tomato slices and avocado and serve.

Nutrition: Calories: 121; Fat: 4.5g; Carbs: 11g; Protein: 9.5g:

Eggs in an Avocado

Preparation time: 15 minutes   Cooking time: 20 minutes

Ingredients:

- 1/2 large avocado, halved and pitted (75g)
- Salt and freshly ground black pepper
- 1/2 tablespoon olive oil (7ml)

- 1 large egg
- 1½ to 2 tablespoons water (30ml)
- 1/4 cup halved cherry tomatoes (37g)
- 2 tbsp chopped fresh chives (6g)

Directions:

1. Place the avocado half, hollow side up, on a clean surface. Flatten the bottom slightly and season with salt and pepper.
2. Heat olive oil in a skillet over medium high heat.
3. Place the avocado half in the skillet, hollow side up.
4. Cook for 1 minute, then crack the egg into the hollow.
5. Season the egg with salt and pepper.
6. Add the water to the pan and cover with a lid.
7. Steam the egg for 3 to 5 minutes until set to your liking.
8. In a bowl, mix tomatoes, chives, and remaining olive oil.
9. Season with salt and pepper.
10. Transfer the egg-stuffed avocados to a plate and top with the tomato-chive mixture.

Nutrition: Calories: 173; Fat: 1g; Carbs: 5.5g; Protein: 4.5g

Shrimp Salad with Avocado

Preparation time: 10 minutes   Cooking time: 10 minutes

Ingredients:

- 1/2 lb. cooked and peeled shrimp (225g)

- 1/2 avocado, diced (75g)
- 2 tbsp minced red onion (15g)

- 2 tbsp minced celery (15g)
- 1 tbsp sliced fresh cilantro (4g)
- 1 tbsp low-fat Greek yogurt (15g)
- 1/2 tbsp citrus juice, fresh (7.5ml)
- Salt and pepper to taste.

Directions:

1. Combine shrimp, avocado, red onion, celery, and cilantro in a bowl.
2. In a small bowl, mix Greek yogurt, citrus juice, salt, and pepper.
3. Pour the dressing over the shrimp mixture and toss.
4. Serve chilled on a bed of lettuce or as a sandwich filling.

Nutrition: Calories: 234.5; Fat: 2.7g; Carbs: 1.8g; Protein: 16.15g

Peanut Butter Banana Oatmeal

Preparation time: 5 minutes

Cooking time: 10 minutes

Ingredients:

- 1/2 banana
- 1/4 cup rolled oats (20g)
- 1/4 cup low-fat milk or plant-based milk alternative (60ml)
- 1 tbsp peanut butter (15g)
- 1/2 tbsp honey (optional) (10g)

Directions:

1. Peel and mash the banana in a saucepan.
2. Add oats, milk, and peanut butter.
3. Cook over medium heat, stirring occasionally, until desired consistency is reached.
4. Add honey if desired.

Nutrition: Calories: 184.5; Fat: 6g; Carbs: 15.5g; Protein: 5.5g

Creamy Millet Porridge with Berries

Preparation time: 5 minutes

Cooking time: 25 minutes

Ingredients:

- 1 cup strawberries (150g)
- 1/2 tbsp maple syrup (7.5ml)
- 3/4 cup almond milk with added protein or soy milk (180ml)
- 2 tbsp sliced almonds (15g)
- 1/2 cup millet (90g)
- 3/4 cups of water (180ml)

Directions:

1. Preheat oven to 375°F (190°C). Mix maple syrup with strawberries.
2. Roast for 15-20 minutes until tender.
3. Toast millet in a pan over medium heat for 3-4 minutes.
4. Let cool slightly.
5. Grind millet, milk, and water in a saucepan over medium-low heat for 15-20 minutes, until porridge-like.
6. Add more milk if needed.
7. Serve topped with extra milk, almonds, and roasted strawberries.

Nutrition: Calories: 280.5; Fat: 6g; Carbs: 4g; Protein: 8g

Apricot Granola with Fresh Fruit

Preparation time: 5 minutes   Cooking time: 5 minutes

Ingredients:

- 2 tbsp gluten-free rolled oats (15g)
- 1 tbsp almonds (15g)
- 1 tbsp walnuts (15g)
- 1 tbsp ground flaxseed (7g)
- 1/2 tbsp olive oil (7.5ml)
- 1/2 tbsp maple syrup (7.5ml)
- Pinch of ground cinnamon
- 2 tbsp chopped dried apricots (30g)
- 1/2 mango, peeled and chopped (100g)
- 1/2 cup fresh strawberries, sliced (75g)
- 1/4 cup fresh blueberries (37g)
- Nonfat dairy milk or plant-based milk for topping

Directions:

1. Toast oats, almonds, walnuts, and flaxseed in a pan over medium heat.
2. Add olive oil and maple syrup, stirring until mixed.
3. Sprinkle cinnamon, add apricots, and combine. Remove from heat and cool.
4. Prepare the fruit and divide the granola into bowls.
5. Top with fresh fruit and milk.

Nutrition: Calories: 189; Fat: 3.5g; Carbs: 2g; Protein: 4g

Smashed Peas, Avocado, and Egg Toast

Preparation time: 5 minutes   Cooking time: 10 minutes

Ingredients:

- 1 slice whole-grain bread, halved (30g)
- 1/4 ripe avocado, sliced (37.5g)
- 2 tbsp peas, fresh or frozen and thawed (15g)
- Salt and freshly ground black pepper to taste
- 1/4 red onion, thinly sliced (15g)
- 1/2 hard-boiled egg, cut in half (25g)
- Fresh basil leaves, for garnish

Directions:

1. Toast bread and set aside.
2. Mash avocado with peas.
3. Season with salt and pepper.
4. Spread on toast, with avocado, onion, egg, and basil.
5. Top equally with the remaining avocado slices, red onion slices, egg, and basil.

Nutrition: Calories: 11; Fat: 6.5g; Carbs: 11g; Protein: 4g

Coconut Milk Pudding

Preparation time: 5 minutes, + overnight chilling   Cooking time: 0 minutes

Ingredients:

- 1/4 cup chia seeds (30g)
- 1 cup light coconut milk (240g)
- 1 ½ teaspoons honey (7.5ml)
- 2 tbsp sliced banana (15g)
- 2 tbsp fresh raspberries (15g)
- 3/4 tbsp sliced almonds (5g)
- 3/4 tbsp chopped walnuts (5g)
- 1 teaspoon unsweetened cocoa powder (2g)

Directions:

1. Combine chia seeds, coconut milk, and honey.
2. Divide into jars and refrigerate overnight.
3. Top with banana, raspberries, almonds, walnuts, and cocoa.
4. Drizzle with honey.

Nutrition: Calories: 366; Fat: 1.5g; Carbs: 0.5g; Protein: 6.5g

Apple Cinnamon Quinoa Breakfast Bowl

Preparation time: 5 minutes

Cooking time: 15 minutes + 5 minutes resting time

Ingredients:

- 1/4 cup uncooked quinoa (43g)
- 1/2 cup unsweetened vanilla or unflavored almond milk (120ml)
- 1 cinnamon stick or 1/2 tbsp ground cinnamon (1g)
- A pinch of salt
- 1 tbsp sliced almonds (15g)
- 1/2 cup sliced apple (55g)
- 1 tbsp hemp seeds (10g)
- Alternative sweeteners: stevia, brown sugar, honey

Directions:

1. Rinse quinoa thoroughly and drain.
2. In a saucepan, combine almond milk, cinnamon stick (or ground cinnamon), and a pinch of salt with quinoa.
3. Bring to a simmer, then reduce the heat to medium and cover. Simmer for 15 minutes.

4. Turn off the heat and let the quinoa sit for 5 minutes to absorb the milk and finish cooking.

5. Divide quinoa into two bowls.

6. Top each with almonds, apple slices, and hemp seeds.

7. Sweeten as desired with stevia, brown sugar, or honey, and serve.

Nutrition: Calories: 180; Fat: 6.5g; Carbs: 7g; Protein: 7g

Spinach & Egg Scramble with Raspberries

Preparation time: 3 minutes

Cooking time: 10 minutes

Ingredients:

- 1/2 cup fresh spinach leaves (15g)
- 1 egg
- Salt and pepper to taste
- 2 tbsp raspberries (20g)
- 1/2 tablespoon olive oil (7.5ml)

Directions:

1. Heat olive oil in a skillet over medium heat.

2. Add spinach and cook until wilted, about 2-3 minutes.

3. Scramble the egg into the skillet, seasoning with salt and pepper.

4. Scramble egg and spinach together until eggs are cooked, about 2-3 minutes.

5. Gently fold in raspberries.

6. Serve immediately.

Nutrition: Calories: 148; Fat: 7.85g; Carbs: 10.45g; Protein: 8.9g

Carrot Baked Oatmeal

Preparation time: 15 minutes

Cooking time: 45 minutes

Ingredients:

- 1 cup dried oats (90g)
- 1/2 cup chopped carrots (60g)
- 1/4 cup sliced walnuts (30g)
- 1/4 cup raisins (30g)

- 1/2 tsp cinnamon
- 1/4 tsp cardamom
- A pinch of salt
- 3/4 cup low-fat milk or plant-based milk (180ml)
- 1/4 cup maple syrup (60ml)
- 1 egg
- 1/2 tsp vanilla extract

Directions:

1. Preheat oven to 350°F (175°C). Grease a baking dish.
2. Mix oats, carrots, walnuts, raisins, cinnamon, cardamom, and salt.
3. In another bowl, combine milk, maple syrup, egg, and vanilla.
4. Stir wet ingredients into dry.
5. Transfer to baking dish.
6. Bake for 35 to 40 minutes until golden brown.

Nutrition: Calories: 118; Fat: 9g; Carbs: 0.5g; Protein: 9.5g

Bagel Avocado Toast

Preparation time: 5 minutes   Cooking time: 5 minutes

Ingredients:

- 1/2 bagel, sliced in half and toasted (45g)
- 1/2 avocado, mashed (100g)
- Salt and pepper to taste
- Optional toppings: cherry tomatoes, red onion, lemon juice, hot sauce

Directions:

1. Toast the bagel halves until crispy and golden brown.
2. Mash the avocado with salt and pepper.
3. Spread mashed avocado on toasted bagel halves.
4. Add optional toppings like cherry tomatoes, red onions, lemon juice, or hot sauce.
5. Serve immediately.

Nutrition: Calories: 115; Fat: 5.5g; Carbs: 15g; Protein: 3g

Southwestern Waffle

Preparation time: 10 minutes

Cooking time: 3 minutes

Ingredients:

- 3/4 whole wheat flour (90g)
- 1/4 cup cornmeal (40g)
- 1 teaspoon baking powder
- 1/4 teaspoon salt (30g)
- 1/8 tsp cayenne pepper (0.5g)
- 3/4 cup low-fat milk or plant-based milk (180ml)
- 1 tbsp melted unsalted butter or olive oil (15ml)
- 1/4 cup minced onion (30g)
- 1/4 cup sliced bell pepper (30g)
- 1/4 cup chopped jalapeno pepper (30g)
- 1/4 cup diced cooked turkey or chicken (30g)
- 1/4 cup grated low-fat cheddar cheese (30g)
- 1 egg

Directions:

1. Combine flour, cornmeal, baking powder, salt, and cayenne pepper.
2. In another bowl, mix milk, egg, and melted butter/oil.
3. Combine wet and dry ingredients.
4. Stir in onion, bell pepper, jalapeno, turkey/chicken, and cheese.
5. Cook in a preheated, lightly greased waffle iron.
6. Serve with healthy toppings.
7. You can use sour cream, salsa, or avocado.

Nutrition: Calories: 103.5; Fat: 6g; Carbs: 8.5g; Protein: 4.5g

Pineapple-Grapefruit Detox Smoothie

Preparation time: 5 minutes

Cooking time: 5 minutes

Ingredients:

- 1/2 grapefruit, segmented and trimmed (100g)
- 1/4 cup pineapple chunks (50g)
- 1/4 banana (30g)
- 1/2 cup spinach (15g)
- 1/4 cup water or coconut water (60ml)

Directions:

1. Segment the grapefruit and set aside.
2. In a blender, combine spinach, banana, pineapple, and water/coconut water.
3. Add grapefruit segments.
4. Blend until smooth.
5. Serve in a glass

Nutrition: Calories: 51; Fat:0.1g; Carbs: 12.6g; Protein: 1g

Pistachio & Peach Toast

Preparation time: 5 minutes   Cooking time: 5 minutes

Ingredients:

- 1/2 slice of whole-grain bread (15g)
- 2 tbsp mashed avocado (30g)
- 1/2 tbsp ripe peach, thinly sliced (30g)
- 1/2 tbsp chopped pistachios (7.5g)
- 1/2 tsp honey (2.5ml)
- Salt and pepper to taste

Directions:

1. Toast the bread to desired crispiness.
2. Spread mashed avocado on toast.
3. Arrange peach slices on top.
4. Sprinkle chopped pistachios.
5. Drizzle with honey.
6. Season with salt and pepper.

Nutrition: Calories: 96.5; Fat: 3g; Carbs: 14.5g; Protein: 4.1g

Overnight Matcha Oats with Berries

Preparation time: 5 minutes

Cooking time: 0 minutes (overnight refrigeration

Ingredients:

- 1/4 cup rolled oats (20g)
- 1/4 cup almond milk (60ml)
- 1/4 cup water (60ml)
- 1/2 tsp Matcha powder (6g)
- 1/2 tbsp honey (10ml)
- 2 tbsp mixed berries, fresh or frozen, (15g)

Directions:

1. In a jar, combine oats, almond milk, water, matcha powder, and honey.
2. Stir well. Add berries and stir again.
3. Refrigerate overnight.
4. Stir again before eating, serve cold and warmed up.

Nutrition: Calories: 186.5; Fat: 0.5g; Carbs: 26g; Protein: 3.5g

Strawberry Peach Smoothie

Preparation time: 5 minutes

Cooking time: 5 minutes

Ingredients:

- 1/2 cup chilled strawberries (75g)
- 1/2 ripe peach, peeled and sliced (75g)
- 1/4 cup Greek yogurt (60g)
- 1/4 cup orange juice (60ml)
- 1/2 tbsp honey (optional)(10ml)

Directions:

1. Blend strawberries, peach, yogurt, and orange juice.

2. Add honey if desired.

3. Blend until smooth.

4. Poor into glasses and serve. Add ice for thicker consistency.

Nutrition: Calories: 110.5; Fat: 0.5g; Carbs: 24g; Protein: 4.5g

Breakfast Parfait

Preparation time: 10 minutes

Cooking time: 0 minutes

Ingredients:

- 1/2 cup unflavored Greek yogurt (120g)
- 1/4 cup granola (30g)
- 1/4 cup fresh berries (strawberries, blueberries, raspberries) (37g)

Directions:

1. Layer 1/4 cup of yogurt in a parfait glass.
2. Add a layer of granola.
3. Top with half of the berries.
4. Repeat layers with remaining ingredients.
5. Serve immediately or chill before serving.

Nutrition: Calories: 106; Fat: 1.5g; Carbs: 20.5g; Protein: 4.5g

Almond Butter & Roasted Grape Toast

Preparation time: 10 minutes

Cooking time: 20 minutes

Ingredients:

- 2 slices of bread
- 1 tbsp almond butter (15g)
- 1/4 cup of red grapes (37g)
- ½ tbsp olive oil (7.5ml)
- Salt and pepper to taste

Directions:

1. Preheat the oven to 425°F (220°C). Spread almond butter on bread slices.

2. Toss grapes with olive oil, salt, and pepper.

3. Roast grapes for 8-10 minutes.

4. Toast bread slices for 2-3 minutes.

5. Top with roasted grapes and serve.

Nutrition: Calories: 109.5; Fat: 5g; Carbs: 14g; Protein: 3.5g

Healthy Bread Pudding

Preparation time: 30 minutes   Cooking time: 45 minutes

Ingredients:

- 2 slices whole wheat bread, cut into cubes (60g)
- 1 cup low-fat milk (240ml)
- 1 egg
- 2 tbsp honey (30ml)
- 1/2 tsp vanilla extract

Directions:

1. Preheat oven to 350° Fahrenheit (175° C).

2. Grease a 1/2 cup capacity baking dish.

3. Arrange bread cubes in the prepared dish.

4. Place bread cubes in the dish.

5. In a mixing bowl, combine milk, egg, honey, vanilla extract, and a pinch of salt. If desired, add raisins.

6. Pour the mixture over bread. Stir gently.

7. Bake for 45-50 minutes until the center is firm.

8. Serve warm or at room temperature. Optionally, add nuts, dried fruits, or spices for flavor.

Nutrition: Calories: 78.5; Fat: 2.5g; Carbs: 12g; Protein: 3g

Muesli with Raspberries

Preparation time: 20 minutes   Cooking time: 0 minutes (refrigeration time)

Ingredients:

- 1/2 cup rolled oats /45g)
- 1/4 cup raspberries (30g)
- 2 tbsp chopped nuts (almonds, hazelnuts, pecans) (15g)
- 2 tbsp dried fruit (raisins, cranberries, apricots) (15g)
- 2 tbsp honey or maple syrup (30ml)
- 1/4 cup low-fat milk or yogurt (60ml)

Directions:

1. Combine oats, raspberries, nuts, and dried fruit in a bowl.
2. In a separate bowl, mix milk/yogurt with honey/maple syrup.
3. Pour liquid over oat mixture and mix well.
4. Cover and refrigerate for at least 30 minutes or overnight.
5. Serve with additional milk/yogurt and fresh raspberries if desired.

Nutrition: Calories: 144; Fat: 3.3; Carbs: 25.5g; Protein: 6.5g

Cannellini Bean & Herbed Ricotta Toast

Preparation time: 5 minutes   Cooking time: 5 minutes

Ingredients:

- 1/2 can cannellini beans, drained and rinsed (200g)
- 1/4 cup low-fat ricotta cheese (60g)
- 1/2 tbsp of chopped fresh herbs (parsley, basil, thyme) (7.5 ml)
- Salt and pepper to taste
- 2 slices of sourdough bread, (60g each)
- Olive oil for brushing
- Optional: red pepper flakes, lemon zest, grated Parmesan cheese for topping

Directions:

1. Preheat oven to 375°F (190°C).
2. Mash cannellini beans in a bowl.

3. Stir in ricotta, herbs, salt, and pepper.

4. Brush bread slices with olive oil and place on baking sheet.

5. Spread bean mixture on bread. Add optional toppings.

6. Bake for 10-15 minutes until heated. Serve hot.

Nutrition: Calories: 160; Fat: 4.5g; Carbs: 21g; Protein: 7.5g

Egg Tartine

Preparation time: 10 minutes

Cooking time: 20 minutes

Ingredients:

- 2 slices of whole grain bread (30g each)
- 2 eggs
- 2 slices of turkey bacon
- Salt and pepper
- Arugula (for spreading) – use sparingly
- Grated Parmesan cheese (optional)

Directions:

1. Preheat the broiler. Fry turkey bacon until crispy.

2. Lightly butter bread slices.

3. Broil bread, butter-side-up, for 1-2 minutes.

4. Crack an egg onto each toast. Season.

5. Broil for 2-3 minutes until eggs are cooked to preference.

6. Top with turkey bacon, greens, and Parmesan. Serve.

Nutrition: Calories: 92; Fat: 1.5g; Carbs: 7g; Protein: 5g

Candied Apples

Preparation time: 10 minutes

Cooking time: 30 minutes

Ingredients:

- 2 Granny Smith apples
- 2 wooden sticks

- 1/2 cups granulated sugar (100g)
- 1/4 cup light corn syrup (60ml)
- 1/4 cup of water (60ml)
- red food coloring (optional)
- 1/8 teaspoon of cinnamon (0.6g) (optional)

Directions:

1. Prepare a baking sheet with silicone mat or parchment.
2. Insert sticks into apples.
3. Combine sugar, corn syrup, and water in a pot. Stir to dissolve sugar.
4. Boil, then simmer for about 10 minutes.
5. Add food coloring or cinnamon if desired.
6. Place on baking sheet. Allow to set for 30 minutes.

Nutrition: Calories: 118.5; Fat: 0g; Carbs: 31.5g; Protein: 0g

Tofu Scramble

Preparation time: 10 minutes

Cooking time: 20 minutes

Ingredients:

- 1/2 block of firm tofu (200g)
- 1/2 tablespoon of olive oil (7.5ml)
- 1/4 onion, diced (30g)
- 1/4 bell pepper, diced (30g)
- 1 cloves of garlic, minced
- 1/4 teaspoon of turmeric (2.50g)
- 1/8 teaspoon of cumin (0.90g)
- 1/8 teaspoon of salt (1.35g)
- 1/8 teaspoon of pepper (0.50g)
- 1 tablespoons of nutritional yeast (optional) (15g)
- 1 tablespoon of chopped fresh parsley or cilantro (optional) (15g)

Directions:

1. Drain and press tofu to remove moisture. Crumble into pieces.
2. Heat oil in a skillet. Sauté onion, garlic, and bell pepper.
3. Add tofu, turmeric, cumin, salt, and pepper. Cook for 5 minutes.

4. Stir in nutritional yeast if using.

5. Remove from heat, add parsley or cilantro.

6. Serve with toast, avocado, or your choice of sides.

Nutrition: Calories: 106; Fat: 7.55g; Carbs: 3.55g; Protein: 8.2g

Raspberry Mousse

Preparation time: 25 minutes

Cooking time: 10 minutes

Ingredients:

- 1 cup fresh raspberries (125g)
- 12 tbsp granulated sugar (25g)
- 1 tbsp water (15ml)
- 1 teaspoon of unflavored gelatin powder (5g)
- 1/2 cup light whipping cream (120ml)
- 2 tbsp powdered sugar (15g)
- 1/2 teaspoon vanilla extract (2.55g)

Directions:

1. Cook raspberries, sugar, and water until thickened. Strain to remove seeds.

2. Cool puree. Soften gelatin in water, then dissolve over heat.

3. Whip cream with powdered sugar and vanilla.

4. Fold puree and gelatin into cream. Chill in serving glasses for 2-3 hours.

Nutrition: Calories: 84.5; Fat: 5.5g; Carbs: 8.5g; Protein: 1g

Summer Berry Parfait with Yogurt

Preparation time: 10 minutes

Cooking time: 0 minutes

Ingredients:

- 1 cup mixed berries (strawberries, blueberries, raspberries, blackberries) (150g)
- 1/2 cup plain Greek yogurt (120g)
- 1/4 cup granola (30g)

Directions:

1. Prepare and slice berries.
2. Layer granola, yogurt, and berries in a glass or dish.
3. Repeat layering.
4. Serve immediately or chill. Optionally, sweeten yogurt or add toasted coconut.

Nutrition: Calories: 260.5; Fat: 7g; Carbs: 43.5g; Protein: 9g

LUNCH RECIPES

Chicken and Pesto Sourdough Sandwich

Preparation time: 10 minutes

Cooking time: 55-60 minutes

Ingredients:

- 2 slices of sourdough bread (60g each)
- 1 tbsp pesto (15g)
- 2 oz. cooked chicken breast, sliced (56g)
- 2 tbsp shredded mozzarella cheese, low-fat (15g)
- 2 tbsp sliced sun-dried tomatoes (30g)
- To taste: salt and pepper

Directions:

1. Spread pesto on one side of each bread slice.
2. Top one bread slice with chicken, mozzarella, and sun-dried tomatoes.
3. Season with salt and pepper.
4. Cover with the other bread slice, pesto side down.
5. Toast in a skillet on medium-high heat for 2-3 minutes per side.

Nutrition: Calories: 195; Fat: 6.5g; Carbs: 15.5g; Protein: 18.5g

Turkey and Spinach Rice Bowl

Preparation time: 5 minutes

Cooking time: 20 minutes

Ingredients:

- 1/2 lb ground turkey (225g)
- ½ tsp olive oil
- 1/2 onion, diced (60g)
- 1 clove garlic, minced
- ½ tsp ground cumin
- Salt and pepper, to taste
- 1 cup cooked white rice (90g)
- 1 cup fresh spinach leaves (30g)
- 2 tbsp diced tomatoes (30g)
- 2 tbsp crumbled feta cheese, low-fat (15g)
- 1 tbsp chopped fresh parsley (optional) (15g)

Directions:

1. Heat oil in a skillet. Brown turkey and drain fat.
2. Add onion, garlic, cumin, salt, and pepper.
3. Stir in rice, tomatoes, spinach, and feta.
4. Cook until spinach wilts.
5. Top with parsley if desired.

Nutrition: Calories: 152; Fat: 3g; Carbs: 12g; Protein: 10g

Two-Mushroom Barley Soup

Preparation time: 10 minutes   Cooking time: 20 minutes

Ingredients:

- 1 tsp olive oil (5ml)
- 1/2 cup sliced carrots (60g)
- 1/2 cup diced onion (60g)
- 1/4 cup chopped celery (30g)
- 2 cups chopped button mushrooms (150g)
- 1/2 cup chopped shiitake mushrooms (75g)
- 1 garlic clove, crushed
- 3/4 tsp chopped fresh thyme (0.75g)
- Salt and pepper to taste
- 1 cup nonfat milk or plant-based milk (240ml)
- 1/2 cup water (120ml)
- 25 tbsp quick-cooking barley (25g)

Directions:

1. Heat oil in a pot. Add vegetables, garlic, and thyme.
2. Cook until mushrooms release juices, then evaporate liquid.
3. Add milk, water, and barley.
4. Simmer for 15 minutes until tender.
5. Spoon into plates and devour right away.

Nutrition: Calories: 15.5; Fat: 3g; Carbs: 2.7g; Protein: 9g

Hearty White Bean and Kale Soup

Preparation time: 10 minutes   Cooking time: 30 minutes

Ingredients:

- 1 tbsp freshly squeezed lemon juice (15ml)
- 1/2 cup well-sliced onion (60g)
- 1/4 cup sliced red bell pepper (30g)
- 1/2 tbsp sliced fresh rosemary leaves (7.5g)
- 1 bay leaf
- 1/4 cup of sliced celery
- 2 garlic cloves, thinly sliced
- 1/2 can of white beans (200g)
- 1 cup packed, stemmed, and finely sliced of kale (70g)
- Salt to taste
- 1½ cups low-sodium vegetable broth (360ml)
- 1/2 tbsp olive oil (7.5ml)
- Freshly ground black pepper to taste

Directions:

1. Heat olive oil in a skillet. Add rosemary, onion, bell pepper, celery, and garlic. Cook until softened.
2. Add beans, broth, and bay leaf. Bring to boil then simmer.
3. Add kale and cook until wilted.
4. Season with salt and pepper.
5. Stir in lemon juice and serve.

Nutrition: Calories: 265.5; Fat: 5g; Carbs: 39.5g; Protein: 17g

Chicken and Rice Stew

Preparation time: 20 minutes   Cooking time: 50 minutes

Ingredients:

- 1.5 oz chicken breast, cut into cubes (45g)
- 1/4 cup sliced carrots (30g)
- 1/2 tbsp sliced fresh parsley (8g)
- 3 tbsp dry long grain brown rice (45g)
- 1 garlic clove, chopped
- 1 cup stemmed and deveined kale (70g)
- 1 tbsp lime juice (15ml)
- 3/4 cups low sodium chicken broth (180ml)
- 2 tbsp sliced onion (30g)
- 2 tbsp sliced celery (30g)

- A pinch of dried thyme
- 1/2 bay leaf (0.1g)

Directions:

1. Combine broth, onion, garlic, celery, carrots, parsley, thyme, and bay leaf in a pot.
2. Simmer for 10 to 15 minutes. Add chicken and rice. Cook until rice is tender.
3. Remove bay leaf. Stir in kale and lime juice.

Nutrition: Calories: 265.5; Fat: 5g; Carbs: 39.5g; Protein: 17g

Fried Chicken Bowl

Preparation time: 10 minutes

Cooking time: 10 minutes

Ingredients:

- 8 oz boneless, skinless chicken thighs (225g)
- 1/2 cup whole wheat flour (60g)
- 1 tsp paprika
- 1/2 tsp garlic powder
- 1/2 tsp onion powder
- Salt and pepper to taste
- 1/2 cup buttermilk (120ml)
- Olive oil for pan frying
- 1 cup cooked brown rice (190g)
- 1/2 cup frozen corn, thawed (75g)
- 2 tbsp sliced tomatoes (30g)
- 2 tbsp chopped scallions (30g)
- Optional hot sauce or BBQ sauce for dipping

Directions:

1. Mix flour, paprika, garlic, onion powder, salt, and pepper.
2. Dip chicken in buttermilk, then flour mixture.
3. Pan fry in olive oil until cooked.
4. Combine rice, corn, tomatoes, and scallions.
5. Serve chicken with rice mixture and optional sauce.

Nutrition: Calories: 296; Fat: 6.5g; Carbs: 24.5g; Protein: 7g

Baked Mustard-Lime Chicken

Preparation time: 10 minutes

Cooking time: 20 minutes

Ingredients:

- 1/8 tbsp black pepper (1.85g)
- 1 garlic clove, minced
- 2 tbsp freshly squeezed lime juice (30ml)
- 2 tbsp sliced fresh cilantro (30g)
- A pinch of salt
- 1/4 tbsp of olive oil (4ml)
- 1/4 tbsp chili powder (4g)
- 1 tbsp Dijon mustard (15g)
- 1 skinless, boneless chicken breasts (100g)

Directions:

1. Preheat oven to 350°F (175°C).
2. Blend lime juice, cilantro, garlic, mustard, olive oil, chili powder, salt, and pepper.
3. Coat chicken breast in marinade and refrigerate for 15 minutes to 6 hours.
4. Bake for 18-20 minutes until 165°F.
5. Serve immediately.

Nutrition: Calories: 94.5; Fat: 2.5g; Carbs: 2g; Protein: 13.5g

Easy Keto Korean Beef with Cauli Rice

Preparation time: 10 minutes   Cooking time: 10 minutes

Ingredients:

- 8 oz ground beef (230g)
- 1 tbsp olive oil (15 ml)
- 2 tbsp soy sauce (30ml)
- 1 garlic clove, sliced
- 1/2 tsp grated ginger (1g)
- 1/2 tsp sesame oil (2.5g)
- A pinch of red pepper flakes (optional)
- Salt and pepper to taste
- 2 tbsp green onions, thinly minced (30g)
- 1/2 head of cauliflower, grated (250g)

Directions:

1. Heat olive oil in a skillet. Cook ground beef for 5 minutes.
2. Whisk soy sauce, garlic, sesame oil, ginger, red pepper flakes, salt, and pepper.
3. Pour sauce over beef and simmer 2-3 minutes.

4. Remove from heat and stir in green onions.
5. Pulse cauliflower in a food processor.
6. Cook separately.
7. Serve beef over cauliflower rice.

Nutrition: Calories: 148.5; Fat: 9.5g; Carbs: 4.5g; Protein: 11g

Chicken with Mushroom Sauce

Preparation time: 5 minutes   Cooking time: 15 minutes

Ingredients:

- 1/2 tablespoon olive oil, divided (7.5ml)
- 1 (6-ounce) skinless, boneless chicken breasts (170g)
- A pinch of salt
- A pinch of freshly ground black pepper
- 2 tbsp chopped shallots (30g)
- 2 ounces button mushrooms, sliced (56g)
- 1 portobello mushroom, sliced (40g)
- 1 garlic cloves, minced
- 2 tbsp dry white wine or low-sodium broth (30ml)
- 1/2 teaspoon flour (1.30g)
- 1/4 cup water (60ml)
- 1 teaspoon minced fresh thyme (5g)

Directions:

1. Heat 1/2 teaspoon olive oil in a nonstick pan.
2. Season chicken with salt and pepper.
3. Cook until 165°F (75° C)
4. Sauté shallots and mushrooms in the same pan.
5. Add garlic, then wine, and scrape the pan.
6. Sprinkle mushroom mixture with salt, flour, and cook.
7. Add water and boil until thickened.
8. Remove from heat, stir in thyme and remaining olive oil.
9. Serve chicken with sauce.

Nutrition: Calories: 164.5; Fat: 5g; Carbs: 6g; Protein: 22g

Asian Chicken Lettuce Wraps

Preparation time: 5 minutes

Cooking time: 20 minutes

Ingredients:

- 1/4 tbsp freshly grated lime zest (1.5g)
- 2 Boston lettuce leaves (10g)
- 1/4 tbsp rice vinegar (3.5g)
- 1/4 tbsp low-sodium soy sauce (4.5 g)
- 1/4 tbsp olive oil (3.4g)
- 1 tbsp sliced peanuts (7g)
- 1 lime, cut into 2 wedges
- 1/4 tbsp dark sesame oil (3.5g)
- 1/2 tbsp chili sauce (8.5g)
- 1 garlic clove, sliced
- 1 (6 ounce) skinless, boneless chicken breasts (170g)
- Olive oil nonstick cooking spray
- 1/2 tbsp grated fresh ginger (3g)
- 1/4 cup fresh mint leaves (10g)
- 1/4 cup bean sprouts (26g)
- 1/4 cup sliced red bell pepper (23g)

Directions:

1. Preheat oven to 350°F (180°C). Mix lime juice, cilantro, garlic, mustard, oils, chili powder, salt, and pepper. Reserve a portion of the mixture.
2. Marinate chicken in the rest. Bake for 18-20 minutes.
3. Slice chicken. Fill lettuce leaves with chicken, mint, sprouts, bell pepper.
4. Drizzle reserved dressing. Top with peanuts. Serve with lime wedges.

Nutrition: Calories: 173; Fat: 7g; Carbs: 5.5g; Protein: 22.5g

Pan-Seared Pork and Fried Tomato Salad

Preparation time: 20 minutes

Cooking time: 20 minutes

Ingredients:

- 2 boneless pork chops (170g)
- Salt and pepper to taste
- 1 cup all-purpose flour (120g)
- 1 egg, lightly beaten
- 1 cup breadcrumbs (110g)
- Olive oil for frying

- 2 green tomatoes, sliced (240g)
- 2 tbsp chopped fresh parsley (7.5g)
- 1 tbsp Dijon mustard (15g)
- 1 tbsp honey (21g)
- 1 tbsp white wine vinegar (15g)
- 2 tbsp olive oil (27g)
- Salt and pepper to taste

Directions:

1. Season the pork chops with salt and pepper. Prepare three shallow dishes: one with flour, one with beaten eggs, and another with breadcrumbs.
2. Dredge each pork chop in flour, dip into the beaten eggs, and then coat thoroughly with breadcrumbs.
3. Heat a generous amount of vegetable oil in a large skillet over medium-high heat. Fry the pork chops for 2 to 3 minutes on each side, or until fully cooked. Drain on paper towels.
4. In the same skillet, fry the green tomato slices for 2 to 3 minutes per side, or until they are golden brown. Drain on paper towels.
5. In a small bowl, whisk together parsley, Dijon mustard, honey, white wine vinegar, olive oil, salt, and pepper to make the dressing.
6. In a large salad bowl, combine the pork chops, fried green tomatoes, and the dressing.
7. Toss gently to ensure everything is well coated.

Nutrition: Calories: 177; Fat: 8g; Carbs: 11g; Protein: 14.5g

Bourbon Steak

Preparation time: 10 minutes

Cooking time: 8 minutes

Ingredients:

- 1 (8 oz) steaks (such as ribeye or strip, trimmed of excess fat) (230g)
- Salt and pepper to taste
- 1 tbsp olive oil (13.5g)
- 1 garlic clove, minced
- 2 tbsp bourbon (30ml)
- 2 tbsp beef broth (30g)
- 1/2 tbsp unsalted butter 7g)
- 1/2 tbsp fresh thyme, chopped (0,5g)

Directions:

1. Preheat your grill or cast-iron skillet over high heat.
2. Season the steaks with salt and pepper.
3. Heat olive oil in the preheated grill pan. Place the steaks in the pan and cook for 2 to 3 minutes on each side for medium-rare, or longer if you prefer well-done.
4. Remove the steaks from the pan and set them aside to rest.
5. In the same pan, add garlic and cook for 1 minute.
6. Take the pan off the heat and carefully pour in the bourbon. Ignite the bourbon using a long-handled lighter or match, and let the flames subside.
7. Return the pan to the heat and add the beef broth. Simmer for 2-3 minutes, or until the sauce has reduced and thickened.
8. Remove the pan from the heat again and whisk in the butter until it melts and integrates into the sauce.
9. Return the rested steaks to the pan, spooning the bourbon sauce over them.
10. If desired, garnish with fresh thyme before serving.

Note: Use a high-quality bourbon for this recipe to ensure the best flavor. Optionally, add mushrooms or shallots to the sauce for added depth.

Nutrition: Calories: 184; Fat: 7.5g; Carbs: 8g; Protein: 13.5g

Fish Chowder Sheet Pan Bake

Preparation time: 15 minutes   Cooking time: 15 minutes

Ingredients:

- 2 fish fillets (such as cod, halibut, or haddock) (150g)
- 1/4 tsp Old Bay seasoning (0.8g)
- Salt and pepper to taste
- 2 tbsp all-purpose flour (15g)
- 1 tbsp butter (15g)
- 1/2 medium onion, sliced (60g)
- 1 garlic cloves, diced
- 1 cup low-sodium chicken or fish broth (240ml)
- 1/2 cup light cream (120ml)
- 1/2 cup of sliced potatoes (60g)
- 1/2 cup frozen corn (75g)
- 2 tbsp sliced fresh parsley (30g)

Directions:

1. Preheat oven to 425 F (220 C). Grease a sheet pan.
2. Season fish fillets with Old Bay, salt, and pepper.
3. Dredge fish in flour.
4. Sauté onion and garlic in butter.
5. Add broth, light cream, potatoes, corn, parsley.
6. Simmer.
7. Place fish on pan, pour sauce over.
8. Bake for 15-20 minutes.

Nutrition: Calories: 206; Fat: 9g; Carbs: 14g; Protein: 16.5g

Maple Salmon

Preparation time: 10 minutes   Cooking time: 20 minutes

Ingredients:

- 2 (6 oz) salmon fillets (170g each)
- Salt and pepper to taste
- 1 tbsp olive oil (15ml)
- 1 tbsp maple syrup (15ml)
- 1 garlic clove, sliced

- 1/2 tsp Dijon mustard (2g)
- 1/2 tsp citrus juice (2g)
- 1 tbsp sliced fresh parsley (optional) (15g)

Directions:

1. Preheat oven to 400°F (200°C).
2. Season salmon with salt and pepper.
3. Mix olive oil, maple syrup, garlic, lemon juice, and mustard.
4. Drizzle sauce over salmon in a baking tray. Bake for 12-15 minutes.

Nutrition: Calories: 132.5; Fat: 6g; Carbs: 7g; Protein: 11.5g

Hawaiian Chop Steaks

Preparation time: 5 minutes   Cooking time: 15 minutes

Ingredients:

- 1 lb sirloin steak, cut into 2 pieces (230g each)
- 2 tbsp soy sauce (30ml)
- 2 tbsp brown sugar (30g)
- 1 tbsp olive oil (15ml)
- 1 garlic clove, minced
- 1/2 tsp ginger, grated (1gram)
- 1/4 tsp black pepper (0.5g)
- 2 tbsp pineapple juice (30ml)
- 2 tbsp green onions, chopped (30g)
- 2 tbsp cilantro, chopped (30g)

Directions:

1. In a shallow dish, combine soy sauce, brown sugar, olive oil, garlic, ginger, black pepper, pineapple juice, green onions, and cilantro to create the marinade.
2. Place the steak pieces in the marinade, ensuring each piece is well-coated.
3. Cover the dish and refrigerate for at least one hour, or up to 24 hours for deeper flavor.
4. Preheat your grill or grill pan to medium-high heat.
5. Remove the steak from the marinade and discard any remaining marinade.
6. Grill the steaks for 3 to 4 minutes on each side, adjusting the time based on your preferred level of doneness.
7. Allow the steaks to rest for a few minutes after grilling before slicing and serving.

Nutrition: Calories: 128.5; Fat: 5.5g; Carbs: 8.5g; Protein: 10.5g

Shrimp Capellini

Preparation time: 10 minutes

Cooking time: 30 minutes

Ingredients:

- 1/2 lb. shrimp, peeled and sliced (225g)
- 4 oz whole wheat capellini pasta (115g)
- 1 garlic clove, sliced
- 1/4 cup of white wine (60ml)
- 2 tbsp low-sodium chicken or vegetables broth (30ml)
- 1/2 lemon, juiced
- 1 tbsp olive oil (15ml)
- 1 tbsp butter (15g)
- Salt and pepper to taste

Directions:

1. Fill a large pot with water, add a pinch of salt, and bring it to a boil.
2. Cook the capellini pasta according to the package instructions until it's al dente. Drain the pasta and set aside.
3. Heat olive oil in a skillet over medium heat. Add the sliced garlic and cook for about one minute, until it becomes fragrant.
4. Add the shrimp to the skillet and sauté for approximately 2-3 minutes.
5. Remove the shrimp from the skillet and place them on a plate.
6. In the same skillet, pour in the white wine, lemon juice, chicken or vegetable broth, and season with salt and pepper. Bring the mixture to a simmer.
7. Return the shrimp and cooked capellini to the skillet, adding the butter.
8. Toss everything together until the pasta is evenly coated with the sauce.
9. Cook for another 1-2 minutes, or until the shrimp and pasta are heated through.

Nutrition: Calories: 239.5; Fat: 8.5g; Carbs: 107.5g; Protein: 16.35g

Chopped Power Salad with Chicken

Preparation time: 20 minutes   Cooking time: 5 minutes

Ingredients:

- 2 skinless, boneless chicken breasts (170g each)
- Salt and pepper to taste
- 1 head romaine lettuce, sliced (250g)
- 1/2-pint cherry tomatoes, divided (150g)
- 1/2 avocado, sliced (100g)
- 1/4 red onion, minced (30g)
- 1/4 cup crumbled feta cheese, low fat (30g)
- 2 tbsp fresh parsley, sliced (30g)
- 1 tbsp olive oil (15ml)
- 1 tbsp red wine vinegar (15ml)
- 1/2 garlic clove, sliced
- 1/2 tsp Dijon mustard (2.5g)

Directions:

1. Season the chicken with salt and pepper.

2. Grill or pan-fry the chicken until it is fully cooked through.

3. In a large bowl, combine the lettuce, tomatoes, avocado, red onion, feta cheese, and parsley.

4. In a small bowl, whisk together the olive oil, red wine vinegar, garlic, and Dijon mustard to make the dressing.

5. Pour the dressing over the salad and toss until everything is evenly coated.

6. Chop the cooked chicken and place it on top of the salad before serving.

7. Top with sliced chicken.

Nutrition: Calories: 170; Fat: 6.5g; Carbs: 21.5g; Protein: 7.5g

Honey Walnut Chicken

Preparation time: 5 minutes   Cooking time: 30 minutes

Ingredients:

- 1/2 lb. chicken breasts, sliced into bite-sized pieces (225g)
- 1/4 cup cornstarch (30g)
- Salt and pepper to taste
- 2 tbsp olive oil (30ml)
- 1/4 cup sliced walnuts (30g)
- 2 tbsp honey (30ml)
- 1 tbsp soy sauce (15ml)

- 1/2 tbsp rice vinegar (7.5ml)
- 1/2 tsp sesame oil (2g)
- 1/2 tsp sugar (2g)
- A pinch of white pepper
- 1/2 tbsp cornstarch (4g) mixed with 1/2 tbsp water (7.5ml) (cornstarch slurry)

Directions:

1. In a small bowl, combine the corn flour, salt, and pepper. Toss the chicken pieces in the mixture to coat them evenly.

2. Heat the vegetable oil in a large pan or wok over medium-high heat.

3. Add the chicken pieces and cook for about 3 to 4 minutes on each side, or until they are golden brown and fully cooked.

4. Remove the chicken from the pan and set it aside.

5. In the same skillet, cook the chopped walnuts for 1-2 minutes.

6. Remove the walnuts from the skillet and transfer them to a separate dish.

7. In a small bowl, thoroughly mix together the honey, soy sauce, rice vinegar, sesame oil, sugar, and white pepper.

8. Pour the honey mixture into the same pan and bring it to a boil over medium-high heat.

9. Add the corn flour slurry and stir continuously for about 1-2 minutes, or until the sauce thickens to a denser, more viscous consistency.

10. Return the cooked chicken and toasted walnuts to the pan and stir to evenly coat the chicken with the sauce.

11. Serve the chicken over steamed rice and garnish with additional sliced walnuts, if desired.

Nutrition: Calories: 157.5; Fat: 4.5g; Carbs: 16g; Protein: 8.5g

Black Bean Risotto

Preparation time: 10 minutes   Cooking time: 35 minutes

Ingredients:

- 1/2 tbsp olive oil (7.5ml)
- 1/2 small onion, diced (30g)
- 1 garlic clove, minced
- 1/2 cup Arborio rice (95g)
- 1 ½ cups vegetable broth (360ml)
- 1/2 can black beans, drained and rinsed (200g)
- 2 tbsp grated Parmesan cheese, low-fat (15g)
- Salt and pepper to taste
- Fresh cilantro for garnish

Directions:

1. Heat the olive oil in a large pan over medium heat.
2. Add the garlic and onion to the pan, cooking until they are soft and translucent.
3. Stir in the rice, cooking for about 2 minutes or until it becomes slightly translucent.
4. Gradually add the broth one ladle at a time, stirring constantly. Wait until each addition of liquid is absorbed before adding the next ladle.
5. Continue to cook and stir the rice for about 18 to 20 minutes, or until it reaches an "al dente" texture.

6. Stir in the black beans and Parmesan cheese.

7. Season the dish with salt and pepper to taste.

8. Cook until the cheese is melted and the beans are heated through.

9. Garnish with fresh cilantro and serve immediately.

Nutrition: Calories: 134; Fat: 4g; Carbs: 18g; Protein: 7g

Cilantro-Lime Chicken and Avocado Salsa

Preparation time: 10 minutes   Cooking time: 12 minutes

Ingredients:

For the chicken
- 1 tbsp minced fresh cilantro (2g)
- 3/4 tbsp freshly squeezed lime juice (11g)
- 1 tbsp olive oil (13g)
- A pinch of salt
- 1/4 tsp ground cumin (0.5g)
- 1 (6-ounce) skinless, boneless chicken breasts (170g)
- Olive oil nonstick cooking spray

For the salsa
- 1/4 cup chopped plum tomato (30g)
- 2 tbsp chopped red bell pepper (15g)
- 1/2 tbsp tablespoon finely chopped onion (7.5g)
- 1 tbsp minced fresh cilantro
- 1 tbsp freshly squeezed lime juice (15g)
- 1/2 small peach, peeled and finely chopped (70g)
- A pinch of salt and pepper
- 1/4 avocado, peeled and finely chopped (50g)

Directions:

To make the chicken:

1. In a medium bowl, combine the cilantro, lime juice, cumin, salt, and olive oil.

2. Add the chicken to the bowl and toss to coat evenly with the marinade.

3. Refrigerate for 30 minutes.

4. Remove the chicken from the marinade and discard any remaining marinade.

5. Heat a large grill pan or nonstick skillet over high heat.

6. Spray the pan with cooking spray.

7. Place the chicken in the pan and cook for 6 minutes on each side or until fully cooked.

To prepare the salsa:

1. In a medium bowl, mix together the tomato, bell pepper, onion, cilantro, lime juice, peach, salt, and pepper.
2. Gently fold in the avocado to combine.
3. Serve the cooked chicken topped with the fresh salsa.

Nutrition: Calories: 183; Fat: 8.5g; Carbs: 7.5g; Protein: 20.5g

Green Beans and Mushrooms Spaghetti

Preparation time: 15 minutes   Cooking time: 15 minutes

Ingredients:

- 1/2 lb. spaghetti, whole wheat 225)
- 1 garlic clove, sliced
- 1 tbsp olive oil (13g)
- Salt and pepper to taste
- 1/2 lb. green beans (225g)
- 4 oz sliced mushrooms (115g)
- 2 tbsp grated Parmesan cheese, low-fat (15g)
- 2 tbsp sliced fresh parsley (30g)

Directions:

1. Cook the spaghetti according to the package directions until it's al dente.
2. Drain and set aside.
3. Preheat a grill or grill pan over medium-high heat.
4. Toss the green beans and mushrooms with garlic, olive oil, salt, and pepper.
5. Grill for 5-7 minutes, or until they are tender and have a slight char.
6. In a serving bowl, combine the cooked spaghetti with the grilled green beans and mushrooms.
7. Sprinkle with grated Parmesan cheese and fresh parsley.
8. Serve and enjoy the delicious blend of flavors.

Nutrition: Calories: 219.5; Fat: 4.5g; Carbs: 40.5g; Protein: 8.5g

Balsamic Rosemary Chicken

Preparation time: 10 minutes   Cooking time: 35 minutes

Ingredients:

- 1/4 cup balsamic vinegar (60ml)
- 1/2 tsp olive oil (2.5g)
- 1/2 tbsp chopped fresh rosemary (1g)
- 1/2 garlic clove, minced
- A pinch of salt
- Freshly ground black pepper
- 1 (6-ounce) boneless, skinless chicken breasts (170g)
- Fresh rosemary sprigs, for garnish

Directions:

1. Combine rosemary, garlic, olive oil, salt, pepper, and 1/2 cup of balsamic vinegar (120ml) in a small saucepan.
2. Heat over medium-low, bring to a simmer, and cook for about 3 minutes until the liquid is reduced by half.
3. Cool the mixture in the refrigerator for about 15 minutes or the freezer for about 5 minutes.
4. Spray a 9-by-9-inch baking dish with cooking spray.
5. Place the chicken in the dish and pour the cooled marinade over it.
6. Marinate in the refrigerator for 30 minutes.
7. Preheat the oven to 400°F (200°C).
8. Take the dish out of the fridge, cover it with aluminum foil, and bake the chicken in the marinade for 35 minutes or until an instant-read thermometer reads 165°F (75°C).
9. Place the chicken on serving plates.
10. Pour the cooked marinade into a small saucepan and add the remaining 2 tablespoons of balsamic vinegar. Cook for 5 minutes.
11. Drizzle the sauce over the chicken and garnish with fresh rosemary before serving.

Nutrition: Calories: 114; Fat: 2g; Carbs: 1g; Protein: 19.5g

Turkey Sandwich

Preparation time: 5 minutes   Cooking time: 5 minutes

Ingredients:

- 2 slices of whole-grain bread (60g each)
- 2-3 slices of low-sodium turkey deli meat (50g)
- 2-3 leaves of lettuce
- 2-3 slices of tomato (30g)
- 1-2 tbsp low-fat mayonnaise or mustard 15-30ml)
- Salt and pepper to taste

Directions:

1. Toast the bread if desired.
2. Spread mayonnaise or mustard on bread slices.
3. Layer turkey, lettuce, and tomato on one slice. Season with salt and pepper.
4. Close sandwich with another bread slice.
5. Cut sandwich in half if desired.

Nutrition: Calories: 127.5; Fat: 5.5g; Carbs: 12.5g; Protein: 14g

Salmon and Summer Squash in Parchment

Preparation time: 15 minutes   Cooking time: 17 minutes

Ingredients:

- 1 tbsp sliced shallot (15g)
- 1/2tbsp freshly ground black pepper (3.5g)
- 1/2 tbsp chopped fresh oregano leaves (7.5g)
- 1/4 tbsp olive oil (4ml)
- A pinch of salt
- 1/2 cup sliced yellow summer squash (60g)
- 1/2 cup sliced medium zucchini (60g)
- 1 skinless salmon fillet (170g)
- 1 tbsp freshly squeezed lemon juice (15ml)
- 1/2 tbsp grated lemon zest (3g)

Directions:

1. Turn the oven to 400°F (200°C). In a medium bowl, combine the lemon juice, yellow squash, shallot, oregano, olive oil, salt, and pepper.

2. Place 2 large parchment rectangles on the work surface with the short side of the parchment closest to you.

3. On 1/2 of one parchment rectangle, set half the zucchini slices lengthwise, overlapping them slightly.

4. Place a salmon fillet on the zucchini, sprinkle with half the lemon zest, then top with half the yellow squash mixture.

5. Fold the parchment over the ingredients.

6. Repeat with the other piece of parchment and the remaining ingredients. To seal the packets, begin at one corner and tightly fold over the edges about 1/2 inch all around, overlapping the folds.

7. Lay the packets on a baking sheet and process for about 17 minutes, or until the salmon turns opaque throughout.

8. To serve, carefully cut the packets open, being careful to avoid escaping steam, and with a spatula gently transfer the salmon and vegetables to two plates.

9. Spoon any liquid remaining in the parchment over the salmon and vegetables.

Nutrition: Calories: 291; Fat: 15g; Carbs: 7g; Protein: 35g

Rainbow Trout Baked in Foil

Preparation time: 10 minutes   Cooking time: 15 minutes

Ingredients:

- Lemon wedges, for serving
- Freshly sliced parsley, for topping
- 1/4 tbs. olive oil, plus more for greasing the foil (4ml)
- Freshly ground black pepper
- 1/2 cup peeled, seeded, and sliced tomato (60g)
- Freshly thyme for topping
- 2 fresh thyme sprigs
- 1 small rainbow trout, deboned (170g)
- 1 garlic clove, minced
- Salt to taste

Directions:

1. Preheat your oven to 450°F (232°C).
2. Cut two sheets of sturdy aluminum foil into rectangles, each three inches (about 7.6 cm) longer than the fish you're using.
3. Brush the dull side of each foil piece with olive oil. Place a trout, skin-side down, on each piece. If trout is not available, consider using a local freshwater fish as a substitute.
4. Open the fish flat and season both sides with salt and pepper. Use simple sea salt and freshly ground pepper for better flavor.
5. In a bowl, mix together chopped tomatoes, minced garlic, and 1 teaspoon (about 5 ml) of olive oil.
6. Season this mixture with salt and pepper, then evenly spread it over the center of each fish.
7. Fold the sides of the trout over the mixture and place 2 stems of thyme (or a local herb like sage or cedar) on top of each.
8. Drizzle each fish with 1/4 teaspoon (about 1.25 ml) of olive oil.
9. Center the fish on the foil before folding the foil loosely around it, crimping the edges to form a packet.
10. Bake the packets on a tray in the preheated oven for 10 to 15 minutes.
11. The trout is ready when it is opaque and flakes easily with a fork.
12. Place each foil packet on a plate for serving.

Nutrition: Calories: 160; Fat: 8g; Carbs: 2.5g; Protein: 19.5g

Sesame-Crusted Tuna Steaks

Preparation time: 5 minutes   Cooking time: 12 minutes

Ingredients:

- Olive oil nonstick cooking spray
- 1/4 tbsp olive oil (4ml)
- 1/2 tsp sesame oil
- 1 (6-ounce) ahi tuna steaks (170g)
- 3 tbsp sesame seeds (45g)
- Salt and freshly ground black pepper to taste

Directions:

1. Lightly spray a baking sheet with cooking oil and preheat the oven to 450°F (232°C).
2. In a small dish, mix together sesame oil and olive oil.
3. Use a brush to apply the oil mixture evenly to the tuna fillets.
4. Pour sesame seeds into another small dish.
5. Press each side of the tuna steaks into the sesame seeds, ensuring all sides are well-coated.
6. Place the coated tuna steaks on the prepared baking sheet.
7. Season the steaks with salt and pepper to taste.
8. Bake the tuna in the preheated oven for 4 to 6 minutes per half-inch (about 1.3 cm) of thickness, or until the fish begins to flake easily when tested with a fork.
9. Serve the tuna steaks immediately after baking for the best flavor and texture.

Nutrition: Calories: 260; Fat: 15g; Carbs: 3g; Protein: 28g

Salmon and Scallop Skewers

Preparation time: 30 minutes

Cooking time: 12 minutes

Ingredients:

- 4 oz wild salmon fillet, cut into cubes (115g)
- 1/2 zucchini, cut into slices (60g)
- 1/2 red bell pepper, sliced into squares (60g)
- 1/2 red onion, cut into pieces (60g)
- 4 button mushrooms
- 1 tbsp pineapple juice (from canned pineapple in 100% juice) (15ml)
- 1/2 tbsp freshly squeezed lemon juice (7.5ml)
- 1/2 tbsp snipped fresh tarragon (0.5g) or 1/2 tsp dried tarragon (0.5g)
- A pinch of dry mustard
- A pinch of salt

Directions:

1. Preheat an outdoor grill. In a small bowl, combine the pineapple juice, lemon juice, tarragon, mustard, and salt to make the marinade.

2. Place the salmon and scallops (assuming they are included) in a resealable bag, pour in the marinade, and seal the bag.

3. Turn the seafood in the bag to coat well. Marinate in the refrigerator for 1 to 2 hours, turning once.

4. Bring a small amount of water (enough to cover the zucchini, about 1 to 2 inches deep) to a boil in a small saucepan. Add the zucchini slices and cook for 3 to 4 minutes, or until nearly tender. Drain and allow to cool.

5. Remove the seafood from the bag, reserving the marinade.

6. On 4 metal skewers, alternately thread the scallops, salmon, zucchini, mushrooms, bell pepper, onion, and pineapple. Brush the skewers with the reserved marinade.

7. Grill the skewers, uncovered, directly over medium coals (or equivalent heat on a gas grill) for 8 to 12 minutes, turning once. The seafood is done when the scallops turn opaque and the salmon flakes easily with a fork.

8. Serve two skewers on each dinner plate.

Nutrition: Calories: 130; Fat: 2.5g; Carbs: 16g; Protein: 13g

Shrimp Scampi with Zoodles

Preparation time: 10 minutes   Cooking time: 30 minutes

Ingredients:

- ½ lb raw shrimp, peeled and deveined (225g)
- 2 garlic cloves, minced
- 2 tbsp butter (use low-fat or substitute with olive oil for a healthier option) (30ml)

- 2 tbsp olive oil (30ml)
- 2 tbsp fresh lemon juice (30ml)
- 1 tbsp chopped parsley (15g)
- Salt and pepper to taste
- 1 medium-sized zucchini, spiralized into "zoodles" (150g)

Directions:

1. In a big pan, cook the butter and olive oil over medium-high heat.
2. When the garlic has a nice smokiness, add it and cook it for 1-2 minutes.
3. Season the prawns with salt and pepper after placing them in the pan.
4. Cook for about 3–5 minutes, or until the shrimp are pink and cooked all the way through.
5. Take the shrimp out of the pan and put them on a plate.
6. Add the lemon juice to the pan and stir it to get any browned bits off the bottom. Process for another 1-2 minutes.
7. Put the zoodles in the pan and toss them with the sauce to coat them.
8. Cook the zoodles for 2 to 3 minutes, until they are soft but still firm.
9. Set the shrimp back in the pan and whisk everything together.
10. Serve the scampi on top of the zoodles and add chopped parsley on top.

Nutrition: Calories: 143; Fat: 7.5g; Carbs: 4g; Protein: 13.5g

Lemon Garlic Mackerel

Preparation time: 10 minutes   Cooking time: 5 minutes

Ingredients:

- 2 (4-ounce) mackerel fillets (115g each)
- Salt to taste
- 1 garlic clove, minced
- Juice of ¼ lemon
- Freshly ground black pepper

Directions:

1. Prepare a baking sheet by lining it with aluminum foil.
2. Place the mackerel fillets on the prepared sheet. Sprinkle them evenly with salt and leave them to sit for 5 minutes. This process helps to firm up the texture of the fish.
3. In a bowl, combine minced garlic and freshly squeezed lemon juice.
4. Add ground black pepper to taste, creating a flavorful mixture.

5. Spread this garlic-lemon mixture evenly over the mackerel fillets.
6. Set your oven to broil and place the baking sheet with the mackerel inside.
7. Broil the fillets for about 5 minutes, or until they are cooked through and slightly golden on top.
8. Serve the broiled mackerel immediately.

Nutrition: Calories: 151; Fat: 10g; Carbs: 0.5g; Protein: 13.5g

Broiled Tuna Steaks with Lime

Preparation time: 5 minutes   Cooking time: 8 minutes

Ingredients:

- Olive oil nonstick cooking spray
- 1 (6-ounce) tuna steak (170g)
- 1/2 teaspoon freshly grated lime zest (1g)
- A pinch of salt
- 1/4 teaspoon freshly ground black pepper (1g)
- 1/2 garlic clove, minced
- Lemon wedges for serving

Directions:

1. Preheat the broiler.
2. Spray the broiler pan with cooking spray to prevent the fish from sticking.
3. Place the fish steaks on the prepared broiler pan.
4. In a small dish, combine lime zest, salt, pepper, and minced garlic.
5. Mix these ingredients well to create a flavorful rub for the fish.
6. Spread the lime-garlic mixture evenly over the fish steaks.
7. Place the pan under the broiler and cook the fish for 7 to 8 minutes, or until it reaches your preferred level of doneness and flakes easily when tested with a fork.
8. Carefully remove the fish steaks from the broiler and transfer each one to a serving plate.
9. Serve the fish steaks with lemon wedges on the side.

Nutrition: Calories: 158.5; Fat: 5.5g; Carbs: 0.5g; Protein: 25.5g

Oven-Roasted Salmon Fillets

Preparation time: 5 minutes

Cooking time: 15 minutes

Ingredients:

- 1 (6-ounce) salmon fillet, halved (85g each)
- Salt and freshly ground black pepper
- Lemon wedges for garnish
- Parsley for garnish

Directions:

1. Preheat your oven to 450°F (about 232°C).
2. Lightly season the salmon fillets with a small amount of salt and black pepper. The amount of seasoning can be adjusted according to personal preference.
3. Place the seasoned salmon fillets on a nonstick baking sheet, or in a nonstick pan with an ovenproof handle. Make sure the skin side of the salmon is facing downwards.
4. Bake in the preheated oven for 12 to 15 minutes, or until the salmon is cooked through and flakes easily when tested with a fork. The exact cooking time may vary depending on the thickness of the fillets.
5. Serve the cooked salmon with lemon wedges and garnish with fresh parsley.

Nutrition: Calories: 56.5; Fat: 2.5g; Carbs: 0g; Protein: 8.5

Moroccan Spiced Chicken with Onions

Preparation time: 15 minutes

Cooking time: 20 minutes

Ingredients:

- 1/2 teaspoon ground cinnamon (1g)
- 1/2 teaspoon paprika (1g)
- 1/2 teaspoon ground cumin (1g)
- 1/4 teaspoon ground cardamom (0.50g)
- 1/4 teaspoon ground coriander (0.50g)

- 1/4 teaspoon ground ginger (0.50g)
- 1/4 teaspoon ground turmeric (0.50g)
- ½ tablespoon olive oil, divided (7g)

- 1 (6-ounce) skinless, boneless chicken breast (170g)
- A pinch of salt
- Olive oil nonstick cooking spray
- ½ cup sliced yellow onion (60g)
- ½ teaspoon honey

Directions:

1. In a small dish, mix together turmeric, ginger, coriander, cumin, paprika, and cardamom.
2. In a large ovenproof skillet over medium-low heat, add 1/2 tablespoon (about 7.5 ml) of olive oil, swirling to coat the pan. Add the spice mixture to the skillet, stirring regularly, and cook for three minutes or until the spices are toasted.
3. Place the chicken breasts in a large resealable bag, add the toasted spice mixture, seal the bag, and shake well to coat the chicken.
4. Season the chicken and then place it in the fridge for ten minutes to marinate.
5. Preheat the oven to 350°F (about 175°C).
6. Remove the chicken from the bag and season it evenly with some salt.
7. Lightly spray the skillet with cooking spray and heat it over medium-high heat.
8. Cook the chicken for about 4 minutes on one side. Flip the chicken and cook for an additional minute. Then remove the chicken from the pan.
9. Add the remaining 1/2 tablespoon (about 7.5 ml) of olive oil to the skillet.
10. Add the onion and sauté for 2 minutes, or until it begins to soften and color.
11. Add honey to the pan and return the chicken to the skillet.
12. Bake in the preheated oven for 10 minutes, or until an instant-read thermometer inserted into the chicken registers 165°F (about 74°C).
13. Serve the chicken immediately after cooking.

Nutrition: Calories: 147.5; Fat: 5g; Carbs: 5.5g; Protein: 20g

Spaghetti Squash and Chickpea Sauté

Preparation time: 5 minutes   Cooking time: 15 minutes

Ingredients:

- 1/2 medium spaghetti squash, halved and seeded (500 g)
- 1 tbsp olive oil (15 ml)
- 1/2 onion, diced (60 g)
- 1 garlic clove, minced
- 1/2 can (7.5 oz) chickpeas, drained and rinsed (215 g)
- 1/4 cup vegetable broth (60 ml)
- 2 tbsp diced tomatoes (30 g)
- 1/2 tsp dried oregano
- 1/2 tsp dried basil
- A pinch of red pepper flakes (optional)
- Salt and pepper to taste
- 2 tbsp chopped fresh parsley or cilantro (optional) (30 g)
- Grated Parmesan cheese for serving (optional)

Directions:

1. Preheat the oven to 375°F (about 190°C).
2. Place the spaghetti squash halves cut-side-down on a baking sheet lined with parchment paper.
3. Roast in the oven for 30 to 40 minutes, or until the flesh is tender and can easily be shredded into strands with a fork.
4. Remove the squash from the oven and allow it to cool for a bit. Once it's cool enough to handle, use a fork to scrape out the spaghetti-like strands from the skin. Set these strands aside.
5. Heat some olive oil in a large skillet over medium heat.
6. Add the minced garlic and chopped onion, and sauté for 2-3 minutes, or until they are soft and fragrant.
7. Add the sliced tomatoes, chickpeas, vegetable broth, oregano, red pepper flakes, basil, salt, and pepper to the skillet.
8. Bring the mixture to a simmer and cook for 5-7 minutes, or until the sauce has slightly thickened.
9. Stir in the spaghetti squash strands and cook for an additional 2-3 minutes, or until everything is heated through.
10. Remove the skillet from heat and stir in fresh parsley or cilantro, if using.
11. Serve the dish with grated Parmesan cheese on top, if desired.

Nutrition: Calories: 122.5; Fat: 5g; Carbs: 13.5g; Protein: 3.5g

Grilled Chicken Breasts with Plum Salsa

Preparation time: 5 minutes

Cooking time: 12 minutes

Ingredients:

For the chicken

- A pinch of salt
- 1/2 tbsp olive oil (7.5 ml)
- 1/8 tbsp ground cumin
- 1/8 tbsp garlic powder

- 1 skinless, boneless chicken breast (170 g)
- 1/2 tbsp brown sugar

For the plum salsa

- 1 tbsp chopped red bell pepper (15 g)
- A pinch of hot sauce

- 1 tbsp sliced red onion (15 g)
- 1/2 cup sliced ripe plum (60 g)
- 1 tbsp cider vinegar (15 ml)

Directions:

1. In a small dish, combine brown sugar, cumin, garlic powder, and salt. The amount of each ingredient can be adjusted according to your taste preferences.
2. Rub the spice mixture all over the chicken, ensuring it's evenly coated.
3. Heat some olive oil in a nonstick skillet or griddle pan over medium heat.
4. Once the oil is warm, add the chicken to the skillet.
5. Cook the chicken for 6 minutes on each side, or until it's well-cooked and browned on the outside.
6. Check the doneness of the chicken with an instant-read thermometer. The chicken is cooked when the internal temperature reaches 165°F (about 74°C).

Nutrition: Calories: 132.5; Fat: 2.5g; Carbs: 8g; Protein: 20.5g

Pesto Pasta

Preparation time: 5 minutes

Cooking time: 10 minutes

Ingredients:

- 1 cup fresh basil leaves (15g)
- ¼ cup extra-virgin olive oil (60ml)
- Salt and pepper to taste
- ¼ cup grated Parmesan cheese (low-fat) (30g)
- ¼ cup pine nuts (30g)
- 1½ garlic cloves
- ½ lb. whole wheat pasta (225g)

Directions:

1. In a food processor, combine the basil leaves, grated Parmesan cheese, pine nuts, and garlic cloves.
2. Pulse the mixture until everything is finely minced.
3. With the food processor running, slowly pour in olive oil through the feed tube until the mixture reaches your desired consistency.
4. Season the pesto with salt and pepper to taste.
5. Cook the pasta according to the instructions on the package. Before draining, reserve 1 cup (about 240 ml) of the pasta cooking water.
6. Drain the pasta and then add it to the food processor with the prepared pesto.
7. Pulse until the pasta and pesto are thoroughly combined. If the mixture is too thick, gradually add the reserved pasta water until you achieve the desired consistency.
8. Serve the pesto pasta immediately, garnishing with additional grated Parmesan cheese and pine nuts.

Nutrition: Calories: 112.5; Fat: 3.5g; Carbs: 16g; Protein: 4g

Chicken Kebabs Mexicana

Preparation time: 30 minutes

Cooking time: 10 minutes

Ingredients:

- 1/2 pound chicken breast, cut into cubes (225g)
- 2 tbsp olive oil (30ml)
- 1 garlic clove, minced
- 1/2 tsp ground cumin (1g)
- 1/2 tsp smoked paprika (1g)

- 1/2 tsp dried oregano (0.5)
- A pinch of salt and black pepper
- 1/2 red bell pepper, cubed (60g)
- 1/2 onion, cut into wedges (60g)
- 6 skewers

Directions:

1. In a mixing bowl, combine olive oil, oregano, cumin, minced garlic, paprika, salt, and pepper to create the marinade.
2. Add the chicken cubes to the bowl and toss them until they are evenly coated with the marinade. For the best flavor, cover the bowl and refrigerate for at least an hour, or overnight if possible.
3. Preheat your grill or broiler to medium-high heat.
4. Thread the marinated chicken cubes, bell pepper pieces, and onion chunks alternately onto skewers.
5. Grill or broil the kebabs for about 8 to 10 minutes per side, or until the chicken is fully cooked and the vegetables have a slight char.
6. Serve the chicken kebabs with optional toppings like sour cream, avocado, and cilantro as desired.

Nutrition: Calories: 83; Fat: 4g; Carbs: 4.5g; Protein: 7.5g

Chicken Cutlets with Pineapple Rice

Preparation time: 10 minutes

Cooking time: 20 minutes

Ingredients:

- 2 boneless, skinless chicken cutlets (170g each)
- Salt and pepper to taste
- 1/4 cup whole wheat flour (30g)
- 1 egg, beaten
- 1/2 cup whole wheat panko breadcrumbs (60g)

Ingredients for Pineapple Rice:

- 1/2 cup diced pineapple (80g)
- 1/2 cup uncooked brown rice (90g)
- 1 cup low-sodium chicken broth (240ml)

- 1/2 tbsp vegetable oil (7.5ml)
- 1/2 tsp low-sodium soy sauce

Directions:

1. Preheat the oven to 375°F (190°C). Season the chicken cutlets with salt and pepper. Coat the cutlets in flour, shaking off any excess.
2. Dip the floured cutlets in beaten eggs, then coat them in panko breadcrumbs.
3. Heat oil in a large pan over medium-high heat.
4. Once the pan is hot, add the chicken cutlets. Cook them for 2 to 3 minutes on each side, or until they are golden brown.
5. Transfer the browned chicken cutlets to a baking tray and place them in the preheated oven. Bake for 10-12 minutes.
6. In a saucepan, bring chicken broth to a boil.
7. In a separate pan, combine rice, diced pineapple, and soy sauce.
8. Reduce the heat to low, cover the pan, and let it simmer for 18-20 minutes, or until the rice is tender and all the liquid has been absorbed.

Nutrition: Calories: 264.5; Fat: 4.5g; Carbs: 36g; Protein: 18.5g

DINNER RECIPES

Oven-Roasted Salmon with Vinaigrette

Preparation time: 5 minutes   Cooking time: 24-25 minutes

Ingredients:

- 2 (6-oz.) salmon fillets (about 170g each)
- Salt and pepper to taste
- 1 lemon, divided

- 1 tbsp olive oil (about 15ml)
- 2 tbsp fresh parsley, chopped (30g)

Directions:

1. Preheat your oven to 425°F (220°C).
2. Season the salmon fillets with salt and pepper.
3. Place the lemon halves, cut side down, on a baking sheet. Arrange the salmon fillets on the same baking sheet.
4. Drizzle olive oil over both the salmon and lemon halves.
5. Roast the salmon in the preheated oven for 12 to 15 minutes, or until it is cooked to your liking.
6. While the salmon is roasting, prepare the vinaigrette. Once the lemons are roasted, squeeze their juice into a small bowl. Add chopped parsley to the lemon juice and mix well.
7. After the salmon is finished roasting, remove it from the oven. Drizzle the charred lemon vinaigrette over the salmon.
8. Serve the salmon immediately, enjoying the added flavor and zest from the charred lemon vinaigrette.

Nutrition: Calories: 161; Fat: 9g; Carbs: 5g; Protein: 16g

Portobello Mushrooms with Mozzarella

Preparation time: 10 minutes   Cooking time: 50 minutes

Ingredients:

- 1/4 tbsp olive oil (about 3.75 ml)

- 3/4 cup diced onion (about 90 g)

- Salt and freshly ground black pepper to taste
- 1 portobello mushroom (about 100g)
- 3 tbsp shredded part-skim mozzarella cheese (22.5g)
- 1/2 cup sliced zucchini (60g)
- 2 portobello mushrooms (85g)
- 6 tablespoons shredded part-skim mozzarella cheese (42g)
- 1 cup sliced zucchini (150g)

Directions:

1. Preheat your oven to 350°F (about 175°C). Line a baking pan with parchment paper.
2. Place a medium-sized saucepan on the stove and heat olive oil over medium heat.
3. Add the chopped onion to the saucepan. Cook for about 20 minutes, or until the onion is soft and browned. If the onions begin to stick to the pan, add a little water and continue cooking until the water has evaporated. Season with salt and pepper.
4. Arrange the mushrooms in the prepared baking pan, stemmed-side up. Fill each mushroom cap with half of the cooked onions and top with mozzarella cheese.
5. Place the sliced zucchini beside the mushrooms in the baking pan. Season the zucchini with salt and pepper.
6. Bake in the preheated oven for 30 minutes.
7. Serve the baked mushrooms and zucchini warm.

Nutrition: Calories: 85.5; Fat: 4g; Carbs: 9.5g; Protein: 5g

Chicken Kebabs

Preparation time: 15 minutes

Cooking time: 45 minutes

Ingredients:

- 1/2 pound chicken breast, cut into cubes (225g)
- 1/2 red bell pepper, cut into squares (60g)
- 1/2 yellow onion, cut into squares (60g)
- 2 tbsp olive oil (30ml)
- 1 garlic clove, minced
- 1 tbsp lemon juice (15ml)

- 1 tsp ground cumin (2g)
- 1/2 tsp ground paprika (1g)
- Salt and pepper to taste
- 6 skewers

Directions:

1. In a large bowl, combine olive oil, minced garlic, lemon juice, cumin, salt, paprika, and pepper to create the marinade.

2. Add the cubed chicken, bell pepper pieces, and onion chunks to the bowl. Toss everything together until the marinade evenly coats all the ingredients. Cover the bowl with plastic wrap and refrigerate for at least 30 minutes and up to 2 hours to allow the flavors to meld.

3. Preheat your grill to medium-high heat.

4. Thread the marinated chicken, bell pepper, and onion alternately onto skewers.

5. Grill the kebabs for 8-10 minutes, turning them frequently, until the chicken is fully cooked and the vegetables have a slight char.

6. Serve the kebabs immediately with your choice of side dish.

Nutrition: Calories: 110; Fat: 1.1g; Carbs: 17.5g; Protein: 7.5g

Indian Spiced Cauliflower Fried Rice

Preparation time: 10 minutes   Cooking time: 10 minutes

Ingredients:

- 1 tsp olive oil, divided (15ml)
- 1 egg, beaten
- 1 garlic clove, finely minced
- 2 tbsp red bell pepper, sliced (about 30g)
- 2 tbsp carrots, sliced (about 30g)
- 2 tbsp onion, chopped (about 30g)
- 1½ cups grated cauliflower (225g)
- 1/2 cup frozen shelled edamame (75g)
- 1/4 tsp ground cumin
- 1/8 tsp ground ginger (0.2g)
- A pinch of ground cardamom and cinnamon
- Freshly ground black pepper
- 1/2 cup fresh spinach, chopped (30g)

- 1 tsp low-sodium soy sauce (5g) (or liquid aminos)
- 2 tbsp cashews, for garnish (about 15g)

Directions:

1. Heat 1 tablespoon (about 15 ml) of olive oil in a large sauté pan over medium heat.
2. Add the eggs and gently stir until curds begin to form.
3. Continue folding the curds over themselves until the eggs are fully cooked and no liquid remains.
4. Transfer the cooked eggs to a plate and break them into small pieces.
5. In the same pan, heat the remaining tablespoon of olive oil.
6. Add the minced garlic and sauté for 30 seconds.
7. Add the chopped bell pepper, carrots, and onion, and cook for 2 minutes, stirring occasionally.
8. Add the broccoli, edamame, cumin, ginger, cardamom, cinnamon, and a few grinds of black pepper.
9. Cook the mixture, stirring frequently, for 5 to 8 minutes.
10. Add the greens and cook for an additional 2 minutes, or until they are wilted.
11. Stir in Bragg's aminos or soy sauce and the cooked, chopped eggs, mixing well to combine all the ingredients.
12. Remove the pan from heat and divide the mixture equally between two bowls.
13. Garnish each bowl with chopped cashews and serve.

Nutrition: Calories: 193; Fat: 11g; Carbs: 14.5g; Protein: 13.5g

Tofu Vegetable Stir-Fry

Preparation time: 15 minutes   Cooking time: 35 minutes

Ingredients:

- 1/2 package firm or extra-firm tofu, drained (about 200g)
- 1/2 cup snow peas (about 60g)
- 1/2 cup sliced red bell pepper (about 60g)
- 1/2 cup broccoli florets (about 60g)

- 1/2 tbsp olive oil (about 7.5ml)
- Ingredients for Sauce:
- 1/2 tbsp rice wine vinegar (about 7.5 ml)
- 1 to 2 tbsp water (15-30ml)
- 1/2 tbsp cornstarch (7.5g)
- 1/2 tbsp grated fresh ginger (7.5g)
- 1 tbsp low-sodium soy sauce (15ml)
- 1/2 tbsp honey (7.5ml)

Directions:

1. In a mixing bowl, combine all the ingredients for the sauce. Set this mixture aside.
2. Preheat the oven to 400°F (200°C). Line a baking sheet with parchment paper or lightly grease it.
3. Arrange the tofu pieces on the prepared baking sheet. Bake in the preheated oven for 25 to 35 minutes, flipping the tofu halfway through the cooking time. The tofu is done when it's slightly firm and golden brown. Once baked, remove it from the oven and let it cool.
4. Heat olive oil in a large pan over medium-high heat.
5. Add the bell pepper, broccoli, and snow peas to the pan.
6. Cook for 5 to 7 minutes, stirring frequently, until the vegetables begin to soften and develop some color.
7. Add the prepared sauce to the pan with the vegetables.
8. Stir well, and the sauce should begin to thicken and bubble.
9. Add the baked tofu to the pan and stir to combine it with the vegetables and sauce.
10. Cook the mixture for an additional 3 to 5 minutes, stirring frequently, until the vegetables are cooked to your preference.
11. Remove the pan from the heat.
12. Serve the tofu and vegetables hot.

Nutrition: Calories: 165.5; Fat: 8g; Carbs: 15.5g; Protein: 10.5g

Pocket Eggs with Sesame Sauce

Preparation time: 5 minutes

Cooking time: 5 minutes

Ingredients:

- 2 large eggs
- 1/2 tbsp sesame oil (7.5ml)
- 1 tbsp low-sodium soy sauce
- 1/2 tbsp rice vinegar (7.5ml)
- 1/2 tbsp minced scallions (7.5g)
- 1 tbsp olive oil (15ml)
- 1/2 tbsp sesame seeds (7.5g)
- 1/2 tbsp dried basil (7.5g)

Directions:

1. In a small dish, combine soy sauce, sesame oil, rice vinegar, and minced scallions. Set this mixture aside.
2. Heat olive oil in a medium nonstick pan over medium heat, swirling to coat the pan.
3. Crack one egg into one side of the pan, and then crack the remaining egg into the other side of the pan. The egg whites will flow together and form one large piece.
4. Sprinkle sesame seeds, cilantro (if using), and ground black pepper over the eggs. Cook for about 3 minutes, or until the yolks are fully set and the egg whites are crunchy and golden brown on the bottom.
5. Carefully flip the eggs with a broad spatula, trying not to break them. Cook for an additional 1 to 2 minutes, or until the whites are crispy and golden brown on the other side.
6. Pour the reserved marinade over the eggs. Gently stir the eggs to ensure the marinade coats both sides, and simmer for 30 seconds.
7. Cut the eggs into slices and serve topped with the pan sauce.

Nutrition: Calories: 120.5; Fat: 9.5g; Carbs: 1.5g; Protein: 7g

Lentil Walnut Burgers

Preparation time: 10 minutes   Cooking time: 10 minutes

Ingredients:

- 1/4 cup chopped red onion (30g)
- 1/6 cup walnuts (20g)
- 2 tbsp packed fresh cilantro leaves (15g)
- 1/2 garlic clove, minced

- A small piece fresh ginger
- 3/8 tsp ground coriander (0.6g)
- 3/8 tsp ground cumin (o.6g)
- 1/4 tsp paprika (o.5g)
- A pinch of salt
- 3/8 cup cooked brown rice (t 45g)
- 1/2 can lentils, divided (215g)
- 1/2 egg, beaten
- 1/2 tsp olive oil, plus a drizzle (2.5ml)
- 1½ tbsp gluten-free oat flour (11g)
- 1/2 cup chopped romaine leaves (30g)

Directions:

1. In a food processor, combine the red onion, walnuts, cilantro, garlic, and ginger. Pulse until everything is thoroughly chopped.
2. Add coriander, cumin, paprika, salt, cooked brown rice, and half of the lentils to the processor. Pulse a few times until the mixture is well combined.
3. Transfer this mixture to a bowl and stir in the remaining lentils.
4. Mix the beaten egg and ½ teaspoon of olive oil into the lentil mixture. Then, stir in the gluten-free oat flour until everything is well combined.
5. Chill the mixture in the refrigerator for 10 minutes.
6. Form the mixture into 4 tightly packed burger patties.
7. Heat some olive oil in a large pan over medium-high heat.
8. Cook the patties in the pan for 4 to 6 minutes on each side, or until they are golden brown and heated through.
9. Divide the chopped romaine leaves equally between two serving plates.
10. Place two burgers on top of the romaine on each plate and serve warm.

Nutrition: Calories: 120.5; Fat: 9.5g; Carbs: 1.5g; Protein: 7g

Zucchini "Spaghetti" with Almond Pesto

Preparation time: 10 minutes

Cooking time: 10 minutes

Ingredients:

- 1/2 cup fresh basil leaves (about 15g)
- 1/6 cup roasted, unsalted almonds (10g)

- 1/4 tbsp sherry vinegar (3.75ml)
- A pinch of salt
- 1/2 medium zucchini, julienned (100g)
- 1/2 tsp olive oil (2.5ml)
- 1 garlic clove, minced
- 1/4 red onion, sliced (30g)
- 1/2 cup green peas (fresh or frozen and thawed) (60g)

Directions:

1. In a food processor, add almonds, vinegar, salt, and ½ cup (about 30g) of basil. Pulse the mixture, frequently scraping down the sides of the food processor, until a smooth paste is formed.
2. Scrape the pesto into a dish and set it aside.
3. Heat olive oil in a medium-sized pan over medium heat.
4. Add minced garlic, chopped onion, and beans to the pan. Sauté for 2 to 4 minutes, or until the onion is translucent and the peas are fully cooked.
5. Add the zucchini noodles to the skillet and cook for 1 to 2 minutes, stirring frequently.
6. Add the previously prepared pesto to the skillet. Toss everything together to combine, and cook for another 1 to 2 minutes, just enough to warm through the pesto.
7. Remove the skillet from heat. Divide the contents between two plates.
8. Top each plate with the remaining ½ cup (about 30 g) of basil leaves.
9. Serve the dish warm.

Nutrition: Calories: 110; Fat: 5.5g; Carbs: 12g; Protein: 5.5g

Farro with Sun-Dried Tomatoes

Preparation time: 5 minutes

Cooking time: 40 minutes

Ingredients:

- 1/4 tbsp olive oil (3.75 ml)
- 1/2 large shallot, diced (30 g)
- 2 tbsp julienned sun-dried tomatoes (30g)
- 2 ounces uncooked farro (56g)
- 1/2 cup low-sodium vegetable broth (120ml)
- 1 to 1½ cups arugula (30-45g)

- 2-3 large fresh basil leaves, thinly sliced
- 2 tbsp pine nuts (15g)

Directions:

1. Heat olive oil in a large pan over medium-high heat.
2. Add the chopped onion to the pan and sauté until it turns golden, which should take about 5 minutes.
3. Add the sun-dried tomatoes and farro to the skillet. Sauté the mixture for about 30 seconds to lightly toast the farro.
4. Pour in the vegetable broth and stir to combine everything.
5. Bring the mixture to a boil.
6. Once boiling, reduce the heat to low, cover the pan, and let it simmer for about 30 minutes, or until the farro is tender.
7. Stir in the arugula and fresh basil into the pan. Cook for 1 to 2 minutes, or until the greens are wilted.
8. Add the pine nuts to the skillet and toss everything together to combine.
9. Serve the dish warm.

Nutrition: Calories: 175; Fat: 8.5g; Carbs: 19.5g; Protein: 6.5g

One-Skillet Quinoa and Vegetables

Preparation time: 10 minutes   Cooking time: 30 minutes

Ingredients:

- 1 tbsp olive oil (15 ml)
- 1 cup chopped sweet onion (200g)
- 1/2 cup chopped red bell pepper (75g)
- 2 cups chopped tomato, with juices (400g)
- 1 cup quinoa, rinsed (170g)
- 1 cup water (240ml)
- 1 cup corn kernels (150g)
- 2 cans black beans, drained and rinsed (each can typically about 400g, drained weight 240g)
- 1 tsp chili powder (2g)

- 1 tsp ground cumin (2g)
- Salt, to taste
- Freshly ground black pepper, to taste
- 1/2 cup chopped fresh cilantro, for garnish (optional) (30g)

- Avocado slices, for garnish (optional)
- 2 limes, sliced, for garnish (optional)

Directions:

1. Heat the olive oil in a skillet over medium heat.
2. Sauté the chopped sweet onion and red bell pepper for 3 to 4 minutes, or until they are softened.
3. Add the chopped tomato (with any juices), quinoa, water, corn, black beans, cumin, chili powder, and salt and pepper to taste to the skillet.
4. Bring the mixture to a boil. Once boiling, reduce the heat, cover the skillet, and simmer for 20 to 25 minutes, or until the liquid has completely evaporated and the quinoa is cooked.
5. Remove the skillet from the heat. Divide the mixture evenly between two plates.
6. Serve warm, garnished with chopped fresh cilantro, and if desired, avocado pieces and a squeeze of fresh lime.

Nutrition: Calories: 266.5; Fat: 5.5g; Carbs: 12g; Protein: 5.5g

Tarragon Sweet Potato and Egg Skillet

Preparation time: 5 minutes

Cooking time: 20 minutes

Ingredients:

- 1 large egg
- 1/2 tbsp dried tarragon (3.75ml)
- A pinch of salt and black pepper
- 1 medium sweet potato, cut into chunks (150g)
- 2 tbsp nutritional yeast or low-fat cheese (15 g)

- 1/4 cup water (60ml)
- 1/4 cup sliced tomato (30 g)
- 1/4 tbsp olive oil (3.75ml)
- 2 tbsp thinly sliced scallions (15g)

Directions:

1. Heat the olive oil in a large pan over medium heat.
2. Add the sweet potato chunks and season with dried tarragon, salt, and pepper.
3. Stir the mixture, cover the pan, and cook for about 5 minutes, stirring halfway through.
4. Add the water and sliced tomato to the pan.
5. Cover again and continue cooking for about 10 more minutes, or until the sweet potatoes are tender.
6. Stir occasionally and add a bit more water (1 to 2 tablespoons at a time) if the skillet starts to get too dry.
7. Once the sweet potatoes are tender, sprinkle nutritional yeast or low-fat cheese evenly over the top.
8. Create two small wells in the sweet potato mixture, ensuring there are still some sweet potatoes at the bottom of each well.
9. Carefully crack an egg into each well.
10. Cover the skillet and reduce the heat to medium-low or low.
11. Cook until the egg whites are set to your preference.
12. Remove the skillet from the heat and sprinkle the top with thinly sliced scallions.
13. Serve the dish warm.

Nutrition: Calories: 218.5; Fat: 5.5g; Carbs: 33g; Protein: 7g

Black-Eyed Pea Collard Wraps with Sauce

Preparation time: 10 minutes   Cooking time: 10 minutes

Ingredients:

For the sauce

- 3 tbsp unsalted natural peanut butter (45g)
- 1 tbsp rice vinegar (15ml)
- 1/2 tsp honey (3.5g)

- 1/2 tbsp grated ginger (7.5ml)
- 1 tbsp water (15 ml)
- Dash of sriracha
- Salt

For the wraps

- 3 large collard leaves, trimmed
- 3 tbsp grated carrots (45g)
- 1/2 cucumber, julienned (50g)
- 1/2 can black-eyed peas, drained and rinsed (215g)

Directions:

To make the sauce

1. In a small bowl, combine the peanut butter, rice vinegar, honey, grated ginger, water, a dash of sriracha, and salt. Mix well to ensure all ingredients are well incorporated and any lumps in the peanut butter are eliminated.

To make the wraps

1. Prepare each collard leaf by trimming the center stem lengthwise to make it more flexible.
2. Spread a spoonful of the prepared peanut sauce on the inner side of each collard leaf.
3. On each leaf, layer one-sixth of the grated carrots, julienned cucumber, and black-eyed peas.
4. To assemble the wraps, fold in the sides of each collard leaf and roll it up like a burrito.
5. Secure each wrap with a toothpick to hold it together.
6. Arrange three wraps on each plate and serve.

Nutrition: Calories: 171.5; Fat: 11g; Carbs: 13g; Protein: 7g

Braised Cauliflower and Squash Penne

Preparation time: 10 minutes   Cooking time: 20 minutes

Ingredients:

- 3/4 tsp olive oil (about 3.75ml)
- 1 garlic clove, minced
- 1/2 tsp dried thyme
- A pinch of red pepper flakes
- 1/2 cup low-sodium vegetable broth (120ml)
- 1/2 cup unsweetened almond milk (120ml)

- 2 ounces whole-wheat penne (56g)
- 1/2 cup cauliflower florets (60g)
- 1/2 cup peeled butternut squash cubes (60g)
- 1/2 cup fresh or canned butter beans, drained and rinsed (60g)
- Freshly ground black pepper

Directions:

1. Heat the olive oil in a medium-sized saucepan over medium-high heat.
2. Add the minced garlic, dried thyme, and a pinch of red pepper flakes to the saucepan. Stir constantly and cook for one minute.
3. Add the low-sodium vegetable broth, unsweetened almond milk, whole-wheat penne, cauliflower florets, butternut squash cubes, and butter beans to the saucepan.
4. Bring the mixture to a boil, then reduce the heat and allow it to simmer vigorously, uncovered, for 10 to 15 minutes.
5. Cook until the pasta is tender, and the liquid has thickened and greatly reduced.
6. Remove the saucepan from the heat.
7. Stir in freshly ground black pepper to taste and allow the dish to stand for 5 minutes.
8. Serve the pasta warm.

Nutrition: Calories: 223.5; Fat: 3g; Carbs: 39.5g; Protein: 9.5g

Mushroom Frittata

Preparation time: 10 minutes

Cooking time: 20 minutes

Ingredients:

- 2 eggs, slightly beaten
- 1/2 tbsp fresh basil, chopped (7.5ml)
- A pinch of salt and black pepper
- 1/2 tbsp olive oil (7.5ml)
- 1 cup chopped shiitake mushrooms (70g)
- 1/6 cup chopped scallions (15g)
- 2 tbsp shredded low-fat Cheddar cheese (15g)

Directions:

1. In a medium dish, whisk together the eggs, chopped basil, salt, and pepper.
2. Set aside. Heat the olive oil in a small nonstick pan over medium heat.
3. Add the chopped scallions and shiitake mushrooms to the pan.
4. Cook the mushrooms and onions for about 5 minutes, stirring occasionally, until the mushrooms are soft.
5. Preheat the broiler.
6. Pour the egg mixture over the cooked vegetables in the skillet. Cook over medium heat.
7. As the egg mixture begins to set, use a spatula to gently push the edges towards the center, allowing uncooked egg to flow underneath.
8. Continue cooking until the egg mixture is almost set, which should take about 10 minutes. The surface of the frittata should be slightly moist.
9. Sprinkle the shredded low-fat Cheddar cheese over the top of the frittata.
10. Place the skillet 4 to 5 inches from the heat source in the broiler.
11. Broil for 1 to 2 minutes, or until the top is set and the cheese has melted.
12. Serve the frittata warm, topped with additional sprigs of thyme and basil.

Nutrition: Calories: 165; Fat: 9.5g; Carbs: 11.5g; Protein: 9.5g

Egg, Carrot, and Kale Salad Bowl

Preparation time: 10 minutes

Cooking time: 20 minutes

Ingredients:

- 1/4 cup uncooked quinoa, rinsed (45g)
- 1/2 cup water (120ml)
- 1/2 cup sliced carrots (60g)
- 2 radishes, sliced
- 1/4 fennel bulb, very finely sliced
- 1/2 medium avocado, cubed

- 1 cup chopped baby kale (30g)
- 1 cup mixed baby lettuce (30g)
- 1½ tsp olive oil, divided (7.5ml)
- 1 tsp lemon juice (5ml)
- A pinch of salt and black pepper
- 1 tbsp tahini (about 15 ml)
- 1 egg
- 1 tsp hemp seeds (about 5 g)

Directions:

1. In a medium saucepan, combine the quinoa and water. Bring to a boil, then reduce the heat to maintain a simmer. Cook for about 15 minutes, or until the quinoa is tender.
2. Transfer the cooked quinoa to a large mixing bowl and let it cool.
3. To the bowl of quinoa, add the sliced carrots, radishes, fennel, cubed avocado, chopped baby kale, and mixed baby lettuce.
4. Drizzle the salad with 1 tablespoon (about 15 ml) of olive oil, lemon juice, salt, and black pepper.
5. Toss everything together to combine.
6. Divide the salad between two bowls. Drizzle each bowl with 1 tablespoon of tahini.
7. Heat the remaining ½ teaspoon (about 2.5 ml) of olive oil in a nonstick skillet over medium heat.
8. Crack the egg into the skillet and fry it over medium-high heat until cooked to your liking, about 3 minutes for over-hard.
9. Place the fried egg on top of the salad in one of the bowls.
10. Repeat with the second egg for the other bowl.
11. Sprinkle each bowl with 1 teaspoon of hemp seeds.
12. Serve the salads immediately.

Nutrition: Calories: 330; Fat: 3.5g; Carbs: 23g; Protein: 11g

Grilled Squash Garlic Bread

Preparation time: 15 minutes   Cooking time: 15 minutes

Ingredients:

- 1/2 medium-sized yellow squash, sliced (100 g)
- 1/2 medium-sized zucchini, sliced (100 g)
- 1 clove of garlic, minced

- 1/2 tbsp olive oil (7.5 ml)
- Salt and pepper, to taste
- 1/2 loaf of whole grain French bread (200 g)

Directions:

1. Preheat your grill to medium-high heat. In a bowl, combine the sliced yellow squash and zucchini with minced garlic. Season with salt and pepper and toss with 1/2 tablespoon (about 7.5 ml) of olive oil to coat.

2. Place the seasoned vegetables on the grill. Grill them for about 8-10 minutes, turning occasionally, until they are soft and have developed a slight char.

3. While the vegetables are grilling, slice the French bread into 1-inch-thick slices. Brush the slices with olive oil and season with salt and pepper.

4. Once the vegetables are grilled to your liking, remove them from the grill. Place the bread slices on the grill and toast them for about 2-3 minutes per side, or until they are nicely toasted. After the bread is toasted, remove it from the grill. Top each slice with the grilled vegetables.

5. Serve the grilled vegetable-topped bread slices immediately.

Nutrition: Calories: 162.5; Fat: 7g; Carbs: 14.5g; Protein: 6g

Turkish-Style Minted Chickpea Salad

Preparation time: 10 minutes

Cooking time: 0 minutes

Ingredients:

- 1/4 cup fresh flat-leaf parsley, chopped (15g)
- 1/4 cup fresh mint leaves, chopped (15g)
- 1/4 cup sun-dried tomatoes, drained and chopped (30g)
- 3/8 cup artichoke hearts, chopped (95g)
- 2 tbsp Kalamata olives, pitted and chopped (15g)
- 2 tbsp red onion, finely chopped (about 15 g)

- 3/4 tbsp tomato sauce, no salt added (1.25ml)
- 1/2 tbsp lemon juice, freshly squeezed (7.5ml)
- 1/4 tbsp olive oil (3.75ml)
- 1/4 tsp paprika
- 1/2 can chickpeas, drained and rinsed (215g)
- 1/4 cup cucumber, finely chopped (30g)

Directions:

1. In a large mixing bowl, combine the following ingredients: chopped Italian parsley, chopped mint, chopped sun-dried tomatoes, chopped artichoke hearts, chopped Kalamata olives, finely chopped red onion, tomato sauce, freshly squeezed lemon juice, olive oil, and paprika.

2. Add the drained and rinsed chickpeas (garbanzo beans) and finely chopped cucumber to the bowl.

3. Toss all the ingredients together until everything is well mixed and evenly seasoned.

4. Serve the salad immediately, enjoying the medley of flavors and textures.

Nutrition: Calories: 275; Fat: 6g; Carbs: 42.5g; Protein: 12.5g

Thai Chicken Salad

Preparation time: 10 minutes

Cooking time: 15 minutes

Ingredients:

- 1/2 tbsp olive oil (7.5ml)
- 1/4 cup red onion, finely chopped (30g)
- 1/2 tsp minced garlic
- 4 ounces chicken breast (113g)
- 1 tbsp lime juice (about 15ml)
- 1/2-inch piece ginger, grated
- 1/2 tsp red pepper flakes
- 2 cups Napa cabbage, shredded (70g)
- 1/2 cup snow peas (35g)

- 3/8 cup carrots, grated (about 40g)
- 1/4 cup red bell pepper, diced (30g)
- 2 tbsp scallions, chopped (15g)
- 2 tbsp fresh basil, chopped (15g)
- 2 tbsp fresh cilantro, chopped (15g)
- 2 tbsp cashews, chopped (15g)

Directions:

1. Heat 1/2 tablespoon of olive oil in a large skillet over medium-high heat.

2. Add the finely chopped red onion and minced garlic, and sauté for 2 minutes.

3. Add the chicken breast to the skillet. Cook for 10 to 15 minutes, or until the chicken is browned and the internal temperature reaches 165°F (74°C).

4. Once the chicken is cooked, let it cool and then shred it.

5. In a small bowl, whisk together the lime juice, grated ginger, and red pepper flakes.

6. Gradually whisk in the remaining olive oil until the dressing is well combined.

7. In a large bowl, combine the shredded Napa cabbage, snow peas, grated carrots, diced red bell pepper, chopped scallions, basil, and cilantro.

8. Add the shredded chicken to the salad.

9. Pour the prepared dressing over the salad mixture.

10. Toss everything together to ensure the salad is evenly coated with the dressing.

11. Divide the salad between two serving bowls.

12. Top each bowl with the chopped cashews.

13. Serve the Thai Chicken Salad fresh and enjoy the blend of flavors and textures.

Nutrition: Calories: 222.5; Fat: 10.5g; Carbs: 16g; Protein: 17.5g

Cauliflower Fried Rice

Preparation time: 15 minutes   Cooking time: 15 minutes

Ingredients:

- 1/2 head of cauliflower, riced (300g)
- 1/2 tbsp olive oil (7.5ml)
- 1/2 small onion, diced (50g)
- 1 clove of garlic, minced
- 1/2 cup frozen peas and carrots (60g)
- 1 egg, lightly beaten
- 1 green onion, thinly sliced (15g)
- 1 tbsp low-sodium soy sauce (15ml)
- 1/2 tsp sesame oil (2.5ml)
- Salt and pepper, to taste

Directions:

1. Use a food processor to pulse the cauliflower florets until they have a rice-like consistency.

2. Heat the olive oil in a skillet over medium heat. Add the diced onion and minced garlic, cooking for about 5 minutes, or until they are soft.

3. Add the frozen peas and carrots to the skillet. Cook for 2-3 minutes, or until they are thawed and warmed through.

4. Push the vegetables to one side of the skillet. Pour the lightly beaten egg onto the other side of the skillet. Scramble the egg until it is fully cooked, then mix it with the vegetables.

5. Stir in the riced cauliflower and thinly sliced green onion. Add the soy sauce and sesame oil, combining everything well until the mixture is evenly seasoned.

6. Season with salt and pepper to your preference.

7. Continue to cook for about 5-7 minutes, or until the cauliflower is tender and the flavors are well combined.

Nutrition: Calories: 136.5; Fat: 8.5g; Carbs: 11g; Protein: 6

Salmon with Creamy Feta Cucumbers

Preparation time: 5 minutes   Cooking time: 15 minutes

Ingredients:

- 2 salmon fillets (200g each)
- 1 tbsp lemon juice (15ml)
- ½ tbsp olive oil (7.5ml)
- Salt and pepper, to taste
- ¼ cup low-fat feta cheese, crumbled (30g)

- 2 tbsp Greek yogurt (30ml)
- 2 tbsp fresh dill, sliced (10g)
- 2 tbsp fresh mint, sliced (10g)
- 1 cucumber, sliced (150g)
- 1 clove of garlic

Directions:

1. Preheat your oven to 400°F (200°C).

2. In a small bowl, combine the crumbled low-fat feta cheese, Greek yogurt, 1/2 tablespoon of olive oil, chopped dill, mint, lemon juice, and a pinch of salt and pepper. Stir well to create a creamy mixture.

3. Place the salmon fillets on a baking sheet lined with parchment paper.

4. Evenly spread the feta and herb mixture over the top of each salmon fillet.

5. Bake the salmon in the preheated oven for 10 to 12 minutes, or until the salmon is cooked through and the feta mixture is golden brown.

6. While the salmon is baking, heat a little olive oil in a separate pan. Sauté the sliced cucumbers and crushed garlic until the cucumbers are slightly softened.

7. Serve the baked salmon with the sautéed cucumbers on the side.

Nutrition: Calories: 280; Fat: 12g; Carbs: 4.5g; Protein: 34g

Chicken Salad with Pistachios

Preparation time: 20 minutes   Cooking time: 30 minutes

Ingredients:

- Olive oil nonstick spray
- 1/2 cup carrots, peeled and sliced (60g)
- 1/4 tbsp brown sugar (3.75g)
- 1½ tsp olive oil, divided (7.5ml)
- Pinch of salt and pepper, divided
- 1 (6-ounce) chicken breast, thinly sliced (170g)
- 2 tbsp scallions, sliced (15g)
- 1/2 tbsp apple cider vinegar (7.5ml)
- 2 tbsp shallot, thinly sliced (15g)
- 2 cups baby arugula (30g)
- 1/2 cup red grapes, halved (75g)
- 1 tbsp unsalted pistachios, chopped (15g)

Directions:

1. Preheat your oven to 425°F (220°C).
2. Coat a 9-by-9-inch baking pan and a rimmed baking sheet with olive oil cooking spray.
3. Place the sliced carrots in the prepared baking pan. Sprinkle with brown sugar, 1 teaspoon of olive oil, and a pinch each of salt and pepper. Toss to evenly coat.
4. Roast the carrots in the preheated oven for 25 minutes, stirring occasionally, until they are tender, and the edges begin to turn golden.
5. About five minutes before the carrots are done, arrange the chicken breast slices on the prepared baking sheet. Drizzle with 1 teaspoon of olive oil and sprinkle with 2 tablespoons of scallions, along with a pinch each of salt and pepper. Toss to combine and arrange in a single layer.

6. Roast the chicken for 6 minutes, turning once, or until fully cooked to an internal temperature of 165°F (74°C).

7. Remove the carrots and chicken from the oven and let them cool slightly.

8. In a large salad bowl, combine apple cider vinegar, thinly sliced shallot, the remaining 1 teaspoon of olive oil, remaining scallions, and a pinch of salt and pepper. Let it stand for five minutes to allow the flavors to meld.

9. Add the baby arugula and halved grapes to the salad bowl with the dressing. Toss to combine.

10. Divide the salad between two serving plates. Top each plate with roasted carrots, cooked chicken, and any juices.

11. Sprinkle each plate with 1 tablespoon of chopped pistachios.

12. Serve the salad warm.

Nutrition: Calories: 131.5; Fat: 5g; Carbs: 11g; Protein: 11g

Tilapia with Tomatoes and Pepper Relish

Preparation time: 15 minutes

Cooking time: 5 minutes

Ingredients:

- 2 tilapia fillets (200g each)
- 1/4 tsp salt
- 1/8 tsp black pepper
- 1 tbsp olive oil (15ml)
- 1 red bell pepper, cored and diced (150g)
- 1/2 red onion, diced (60g)
- 1 clove of garlic, minced
- 1/2 pint cherry tomatoes, halved (150g)
- 1 tbsp red wine vinegar (15ml)
- 1/2 tbsp honey (10g)
- 1 tbsp chopped fresh parsley or cilantro (5g)

Directions:

1. Season the tilapia fillets with salt and pepper.

2. Heat 1 tablespoon of olive oil in a skillet over medium-high heat.

3. Add the tilapia fillets to the skillet and cook for 2-3 minutes on each side, or until the fish is cooked through and flaky.

4. Remove the tilapia from the skillet and set aside, keeping them warm.

5. In the same skillet, add the diced onion, minced garlic, and diced red bell peppers. Cook the vegetables for 5-6 minutes, or until they are soft.

6. Stir in the honey and red wine vinegar.

7. Add the halved cherry tomatoes to the skillet. Cook for an additional 2 to 3 minutes, or until the tomatoes are slightly softened and heated through.

8. Stir in the chopped parsley or cilantro.

9. To serve, place the tilapia fillets on plates and top each fillet with the pepper and tomato relish.

Nutrition: Calories: 193; Fat: 3g; Carbs: 0.5g; Protein: 4g

Simple Tomato Basil Soup

Preparation time: 5 minutes   Cooking time: 10 minutes

Ingredients:

- 1/2 cup sliced onion (60g)
- 2 garlic cloves
- 1/2 tbsp olive oil (7.5ml)
- 3.5 cups sliced fresh tomatoes (525g)
- 1/4 cup sliced fresh basil leaves (15g)

Directions:

1. Heat the olive oil in an iron saucepan over medium heat.

2. Add the sliced onion and garlic cloves to the pan. Cook for a minute or two until they begin to soften.

3. Stir in the sliced fresh tomatoes.

4. Cook the tomatoes, stirring occasionally, until they have softened and broken down.

5. Remove the saucepan from the heat. Stir in the fresh basil leaves, and season with salt and pepper to taste.

6. Blend the mixture until smooth using a mixer or an immersion blender.

7. Serve the soup immediately.

Nutrition: Calories: 84.5; Fat: 2g; Carbs: 16.5g; Protein: 3.5g

Creamy Chicken and Chickpea Salad

Preparation time: 10 minutes

Cooking time: 0 minutes

Ingredients:

- 1/2 cup cubed cooked chicken breast (60g)
- 1/2 can chickpeas, drained and rinsed (100g)
- 1/2 cup chopped seeded cucumber (60g)
- 2 tbsp chopped scallions (15g)
- 1 tbsp chopped fresh mint (5g)
- 1/2 garlic clove, minced
- 2 tbsp plain nonfat Greek yogurt (30ml)
- 1 cup baby spinach leaves (30g)
- 1 tbsp sliced almonds (15g)
- 1/2 lemon, cut into wedges
- 1/2 medium tomato, cut into wedges (60g)

Directions:

1. In a bowl, combine the cubed cooked chicken breast, chickpeas, chopped cucumber, scallions, mint, minced garlic, and Greek yogurt. Season with salt to taste and toss gently to combine all the ingredients.
2. Gently fold in the baby spinach leaves, taking care not to bruise them.
3. Divide the salad evenly between two serving plates. Top each serving with sliced almonds.
4. Place lemon and tomato wedges on the side of each plate.
5. Serve the salad immediately. Diners can squeeze the lemon wedges over their salads as desired.

Nutrition: Calories: 195; Fat: 4g; Carbs: 21g; Protein: 20.5g

Seared Tilapia with Spiralized Zucchini

Preparation time: 10 minutes

Cooking time: 25 minutes

Ingredients:

- 2 Tilapia fillets (200g each)
- 1 clove of garlic, sliced

- 1 tbsp butter (15g)
- Salt and pepper, to taste
- 1 tbsp of olive oil (15ml)
- 1/2 zucchini, spiralized (100g)
- Lemon wedges for serving

Directions:

1. Season both sides of the Tilapia fillets with salt and pepper.
2. Heat the olive oil in a large skillet over medium-high heat. Add the Tilapia fillets and cook for 3–4 minutes on each side, or until they are thoroughly cooked and golden brown.
3. Remove the Tilapia from the skillet and set aside.
4. In the same skillet, add the spiralized zucchini, sliced garlic, and butter. Cook for 2-3 minutes or until the zucchini noodles are crisp yet tender.
5. Return the Tilapia to the skillet with the zucchini noodles. Cook for an additional 1-2 minutes, or until everything is heated through.
6. Serve the Tilapia and zucchini noodles with lemon wedges on the side.

Nutrition:144.5; Fat: 6.5g; Carbs: 3.5g; Protein: 18g

Broccoli and Gold Potato Soup

Preparation time: 10 minutes   Cooking time: 35 minutes

Ingredients:

- 1/2 cup of sliced onion (60 g)
- 1 garlic clove, minced
- 1 tbsp olive oil (15 ml)
- 1½ broccoli florets (150 g)
- 1 tbsp dried thyme (7g)
- 1/4 tsp red pepper flakes (0.5 g)
- 1½ low-sodium vegetable broth (360 ml)
- 1 cup of peeled and chopped Yukon gold potatoes (200 g)
- Ground black pepper, to taste
- 2 tbsp of sliced fresh chives (8 g)

Directions:

1. Heat the olive oil in a saucepan over medium heat. Add the sliced onion and minced garlic.
2. Cook for 4 or 5 minutes, until fragrant and translucent.

3. Add the vegetable broth and chopped Yukon gold potatoes to the saucepan. Cover and bring to a boil. Reduce the heat to medium and cook for about 15 minutes.

4. Add the broccoli florets, dried thyme, and red pepper flakes to the saucepan. Cover and steam for 5 minutes, or until the broccoli is tender but still bright green.

5. Transfer the soup to a blender. Season with salt and ground black pepper to taste, and blend until smooth.

6. Ladle the soup into bowls. Garnish each bowl with sliced fresh chives.

7. Serve the soup warm.

Nutrition: Calories: 150; Fat: 4g; Carbs: 24g; Protein: 6g

Braised Lentils and Vegetables

Preparation time: 15 minutes

Cooking time: 60 minutes

Ingredients:

- 1½ olive oil (7.5ml)
- 1/2 diced onion (75g)
- 1 garlic clove, minced
- 1/2 celery stalk, thinly sliced
- 1/2 cup baby carrots (60g)
- 1/3 cup sliced mushrooms (30g)
- 1/2 fennel bulb, cut into wedges
- 1/2 cup dried green French lentils, rinsed and drained (100g)

- 1/4 cup water (60ml)
- 3/4 cup unsalted vegetable stock (180ml)
- 1 fresh thyme sprig
- 1 fresh rosemary sprig
- Salt and pepper, to taste
- Fresh parsley, for garnish

Directions:

1. Heat a deep 4-quart saucepan over medium-high heat. Add the olive oil and heat for 20 to 30 seconds.

2. Add the diced onion to the saucepan. Reduce the heat to medium and continue to cook for about 5 minutes, or until the onion begins to soften and turn brown.

3. Add the minced garlic and thinly sliced celery to the saucepan. Stir periodically and cook for an additional five minutes.

4. Add the baby carrots, sliced mushrooms, fennel wedges, rinsed lentils, and water to the saucepan.

5. Stir and cook for 2 to 3 minutes, until the water is completely absorbed.

6. Add the unsalted vegetable stock, fresh rosemary, and thyme to the pan.

7. Reduce the heat to medium-low, cover the saucepan, and simmer gently.

8. Cook the lentils for 40 to 45 minutes, or until they are tender but not mushy and have mostly absorbed the liquid.

9. Season with salt and pepper to taste.

10. Serve the braised lentils and vegetables garnished with fresh parsley.

Nutrition: Calories: 230; Fat: 3g; Carbs: 38g; Protein: 14g

Acorn Squash Stuffed with White Beans

Preparation time: 10 minutes   Cooking time: 25 minutes

Ingredients:

- 1 medium acorn squash, halved and seeded (700-900g)
- 1/8 tsp salt (1g)
- 1/4 tsp black pepper (1g)
- 1 tbsp olive oil (15ml)
- 1 cup sliced onion (30g)
- 1/2 cup canned white beans, rinsed and drained (120g)
- 1 tbsp wheat germ (7g)
- 1 garlic clove, minced
- 1 tbsp water (15ml)
- 1 tbsp dried basil (3g)
- 1 tbsp dried rosemary (3)
- 5 cups chopped kale (134g)
- 1 tbsp tomato paste, no salt added (15g)
- 1 tbsp feta cheese (15g)

Directions:

1. Preheat your oven's broiler. Arrange the rack in the middle position.

2. To ensure the acorn squash halves sit flat, slice a small portion off the bottom of each half. Brush the inside of each half with 1/2 teaspoon (about 2.5 ml) of olive oil. Season with salt and 1/8 teaspoon (0.5g) of black pepper.

3. Place the squash halves cut-side up in a microwave-safe dish. Cover with plastic wrap and microwave on high for about 12 minutes (check for fork-tenderness).

4. In the meantime, heat 1 teaspoon (about 5 ml) of olive oil in a skillet over medium heat. Add the sliced onion and cook for 2-3 minutes, or until it starts to brown. Add the minced garlic and cook for an additional minute, stirring frequently.

5. Stir in the tomato paste, 1 tablespoon (15 ml) of water, and the remaining black pepper. Add the kale and white beans. Cover and cook for 3-5 minutes until the kale wilts. Uncover and cook for 2 more minutes. Remove from heat.

6. In a small bowl, combine the wheat germ, dried basil, dried rosemary, and feta cheese with the remaining olive oil (1 teaspoon or about 5 ml).

7. Spoon the kale and bean mixture into the squash halves. Place them on a baking tray.

8. Sprinkle the wheat germ and feta mixture over the stuffed squash. Broil for 1-2 minutes or until the topping is golden brown.

9. Serve the stuffed acorn squash warm.

Nutrition: Calories: 250; Fat: 6g; Carbs: 45g; Protein: 10g

Cheesy Artichoke Toasts

Preparation time: 10 minutes

Cooking time: 15 minutes

Ingredients:

- 1/2 can artichoke hearts, drained and chopped (200g)
- 2 tbsp low-fat mayonnaise (30g)
- 2 tbsp low-fat sour cream (30g)
- 2 tbsp (15g) grated Parmesan cheese
- 1 garlic clove, minced
- 1/8 tsp salt (1.30g)
- 1/8 tsp black pepper (0.40g)
- 1/2 baguette sliced into 1/2-inch thick slices (150g)
- 1/2 cup shredded low-fat mozzarella cheese (60g)

Directions:

1. Preheat your oven to 425°F (220°C).

2. In a mixing bowl, combine the chopped artichoke hearts, low-fat mayonnaise, sour cream, grated Parmesan cheese, minced garlic, salt, and black pepper.

3. Mix well to create a uniform artichoke spread.

4. Arrange the baguette slices on a baking sheet.

5. Spread the artichoke mixture evenly onto each baguette slice.

6. Sprinkle shredded low-fat mozzarella cheese over the artichoke mixture on each slice.

7. Bake in the preheated oven for 10 to 12 minutes, or until the toasts are golden brown and the cheese is melted and bubbly.

8. For additional flavor, consider adding other ingredients like chopped parsley, green onion, or a pinch of red pepper flakes to the artichoke mixture before baking.

Nutrition: Calories: 200; Fat: 5g; Carbs: 30g; Protein: 10g

Spring Minestrone Soup

Preparation time: 20 minutes   Cooking time: 40 minutes

Ingredients:

- 1/2 tbsp) olive oil (7.5ml
- 1/2 onion, diced (50g)
- 1 garlic clove, minced
- 1/2 cup diced carrotsn (60g)
- 1/2 cup diced celery (60g)
- 1/2 cup diced potatoes (75g)
- 1/2 cup green peas (70g)
- 1/2 cup corn (70g)
- 2 cups low-sodium chicken or vegetable broth (480ml)
- 1 cup wáter (240ml)
- 1/2 can diced tomatoes (200g)
- 1/2 tsp dried basil (0.9g)
- 1/2 tsp dried oregano (0.9g)
- Salt and pepper to taste
- 1/2 can cannellini beans, drained and rinsed (200g)
- 1/4 cup small pasta (30g)
- 1 cup chopped spinach or kale (67g)
- 2 tbsp grated Parmesan cheese (10g) (optional)

Directions:

1. Heat the olive oil in a pot over medium heat.

2. Add the diced onion and minced garlic, cooking for about 5 minutes or until tender.

3. Add salt, pepper, chicken or vegetable broth, diced tomatoes, water, dried basil, dried oregano, diced potatoes, diced carrots, diced celery, green peas, and corn to the pot.

4. Bring the mixture to a boil.

5. Once boiling, reduce the heat and simmer for 15 minutes, or until the vegetables are soft.

6. Stir in the cannellini beans, small pasta, and chopped spinach or kale.

7. Continue cooking for another 8-10 minutes, or until the pasta is cooked.

8. Ladle the soup into bowls. If desired, sprinkle each serving with grated Parmesan cheese.

9. Serve the soup hot.

Nutrition: Calories: 300; Fat: 6g; Carbs: 45g; Protein: 18g

Lemon-Thyme Chicken

Preparation time: 5 minutes

Cooking time: 20 minutes

Ingredients:

- 2 boneless chicken breasts (400g)
- 1 tbsp fresh thyme leaves (15ml)
- 1 tbsp fresh lemon juice (15ml)
- 2 tbsp low-sodium chicken broth (30ml)
- Salt and pepper to taste
- 1 tbsp olive oil (15ml)
- 1 garlic clove, minced

Directions:

1. Season the chicken breasts with salt and pepper.

2. Heat the olive oil in a large skillet over medium-high heat.

3. Add the chicken breasts to the skillet. Cook for 5 to 6 minutes on each side, or until they are golden brown and cooked through.

4. Remove the chicken from the skillet and set aside.

5. Add the fresh thyme leaves and minced garlic to the same skillet.

6. Cook for 1 to 2 minutes, or until the ingredients become aromatic.

7. Stir in the low-sodium chicken broth and fresh lemon juice. Allow the mixture to simmer for a short while.
8. Return the chicken to the skillet and spoon the sauce over the chicken.
9. Cook for an additional 2 to 3 minutes, or until the chicken is thoroughly heated and the sauce has slightly thickened.
10. If desired, garnish with extra thyme leaves and lemon wedges before serving.

Nutrition: Calories: 250; Fat: 10g; Carbs: 3g; Protein: 35

Roasted Garlic and Tomato Lentil Salad

Preparation time: 15 minutes   Cooking time: 30 minutes

Ingredients:

- 1/2 garlic bulb
- 1/2 tbsp olive oil for garlic (7.5ml), plus 1 tbsp for dressing (15ml)
- 3/4 cup halved grape tomatoes (150g)
- 1/4 cup sliced red onion (60g)
- Salt and pepper, to taste
- 1 cup low-sodium vegetable broth (240ml)
- 1/2 cup green lentils (100g)
- 1/4 cup diced red bell pepper (60g)
- 1/4 cup diced celery (30g)
- 1/4 cup pumpkin seeds (30g)
- 1/4 cup fresh parsley, chopped (15g)
- 1 tbsp lemon juice (15ml)

Directions:

1. Preheat the oven to 375°F (190°C). Line a baking sheet with parchment paper.
2. Cut the top off the garlic bulb. Place the bulb on a small piece of aluminum foil, drizzle with 1/2 tablespoon (7.5ml) of olive oil and wrap the foil around the garlic.
3. Place the halved grape tomatoes and sliced red onion on the prepared baking sheet. Drizzle with 1 teaspoon (about 5ml) of olive oil and season with salt and pepper.
4. Bake the vegetables and wrapped garlic for 25 to 30 minutes, or until the vegetables are slightly shriveled and the garlic is soft.

5. Meanwhile, bring the vegetable broth to a boil in a large saucepan. Add the green lentils, reduce the heat, cover, and simmer for 20 to 25 minutes, or until the lentils are tender. Drain any excess liquid and transfer the lentils to a bowl.

6. Once the garlic is cool enough to handle, gently squeeze the cloves out of the bulb and mash them into smaller pieces in a small bowl.

7. Add the roasted garlic, baked tomatoes and onion, diced bell pepper, diced celery, pumpkin seeds, and chopped parsley to the lentils.

8. In a small bowl, whisk together the lemon juice, remaining 1 tablespoon (15ml) of olive oil, and additional seasonings like red pepper flakes. Season with salt and pepper.

9. Toss the dressing with the lentil salad mixture.

10. Serve the salad, optionally garnished with more fresh parsley or lemon wedges.

Nutrition: Calories: 184; Fat: 10.5g; Carbs: 16.5g; Protein: 8g

Grilled Chicken and Cherry Salad

Preparation time: 30 minutes   Cooking time: 10 minutes

Ingredients:

- 2 skinless, boneless chicken breasts (200g each)
- Salt and pepper, to taste
- 1 tbsp olive oil (15ml)
- 2 tbsp balsamic vinegar (30ml)
- 2 garlic cloves, chopped
- 1/4 cup fresh basil, minced (15g)
- 1 cup fresh cherries, pitted (150g)
- 2 cups mixed greens (150g)
- 1/4 cup feta cheese, low-fat (30g)

Directions:

1. Season the chicken breasts with salt and pepper.

2. Preheat the grill to medium-high heat. Grill the chicken for 6 to 8 minutes on each side, or until fully cooked through.

3. In a small bowl, whisk together the minced basil, chopped garlic, balsamic vinegar, and olive oil to create a dressing.

4. Once the chicken is cooked, allow it to cool slightly, then slice it.

5. On a serving platter or individual plates, arrange the mixed greens. Top with the sliced chicken, pitted cherries, and crumbled feta cheese.
6. Drizzle the balsamic dressing over the salad just before serving.

Nutrition: Calories: 271.5; Fat: 12g; Carbs: 18g; Protein: 25g

Creamy Asparagus Pea Soup

Preparation time: 5 minutes   Cooking time: 25 minutes

Ingredients:

For the soup

- 1/2 large bundle asparagus, trimmed
- 1 tsp olive oil for asparagus (5ml), plus 2 tsp for sauté (10ml)
- Salt and pepper, to taste
- 2 garlic cloves, minced
- 1/3 cup thinly sliced shallots (40g)
- 1/2 cup fresh or frozen peas (120g)
- 1 ½ cups plain soy milk (360ml)
- 1 ½ cups low-sodium vegetable broth (360ml)

For the garlic herb croutons

- 1/8 tsp garlic powder (2g)
- 1 tbsp olive oil (15ml)
- 1/8 tsp pepper (2g)
- 1 cup cubed whole-grain bread (60g)
- 1/8 tsp dried oregano (0.5g)
- 1/8 tsp dried basil (0.5g)
- Grated parmesan cheese, for topping (optional)

Directions:

1. To make the soup
2. Preheat the oven to 400°F (200°C).
3. Arrange the asparagus on a baking sheet. Drizzle with 1 teaspoon (5ml) of olive oil and season with salt and pepper. Toss to coat.
4. Roast in the oven for 15 minutes. After roasting, remove and set aside. Reduce the oven temperature to 325°F (163°C) for croutons.

5. In a large saucepan, heat 2 teaspoons (10ml) of olive oil over medium heat. Add the shallots and garlic, cooking for 2 to 3 minutes until translucent and fragrant.

6. Add the peas, soy milk, and vegetable broth to the saucepan. Season with salt and pepper to taste. Bring to a boil, then reduce the heat and simmer for 5 minutes.

7. Blend the broth mixture and roasted asparagus in a blender until smooth and creamy. Return the soup to the saucepan and heat through.

8. To make the garlic herb croutons

9. In a large mixing bowl, toss the cubed bread. In a small dish, combine the olive oil, pepper, garlic powder, oregano, and basil. Drizzle this mixture over the bread cubes, tossing to coat evenly.

10. Spread the bread cubes in a single layer on a baking sheet. Bake for 15 to 20 minutes at 325°F (163°C), stirring after 10 minutes, until golden brown.

11. To serve, ladle the soup into bowls. Top with freshly ground black pepper, garlic herb croutons, and optional Parmesan cheese.

Nutrition: Calories: 196.5; Fat: 8.5g; Carbs: 22g; Protein: 10g

Pork Fried Rice

Preparation time: 15 minutes   Cooking time: 20 minutes

Ingredients:

- 1 cup (about 200g) cooked brown rice, cooled
- 1/4 lb. (about 115g) lean pork, sliced into small pieces
- 1/2 tbsp (7.5ml) olive oil
- 1/4 cup (30g) frozen peas
- 1 egg, beaten

- 1 ½ tbsp (22.5ml) low-sodium soy sauce
- 1 tbsp (15ml) oyster sauce
- 1 clove garlic, minced
- 1/4 cup (30g) minced onions
- 1/4 cup (30g) chopped carrots
- 1/2 tsp (2.5ml) sesame oil
- Salt and pepper to taste

Directions:

1. Heat a pan over medium-high heat and add the olive oil.
2. Add the pork and cook for 5 - 7 minutes, or until browned.

3. Add the minced garlic, onions, chopped carrots, and frozen peas to the pan. Cook for about 5-7 minutes, or until the vegetables are softened.

4. Push the pork and vegetables to the side of the pan. Pour in the beaten egg on the cleared side of the pan. Scramble the eggs until cooked through.

5. Add the cooked rice to the skillet with the pork and vegetables. Toss everything together.

6. Pour in the low-sodium soy sauce, oyster sauce, and sesame oil over the rice. Stir well to coat the rice evenly with the sauce.

7. Season with salt and pepper to taste. Serve the pork fried rice warm.

Nutrition: Calories: 358.5; Fat: 7g; Carbs: 45g; Protein: 24g

Chicken Satay

Preparation time: 30 minutes   Cooking time: 10 minutes

Ingredients:

- 1/2 lb. (230g) skinless, boneless chicken breasts
- 1/2 cup (120ml) light coconut milk
- 1 tbsp (15g) brown sugar
- 1 ½ tbsp (22.5ml) low-sodium soy sauce

- 1/2 tsp ground cumin (0.9g)
- 1/2 tsp ground coriander (0.9g)
- 1/2 tsp turmeric (0.9g)
- 1/4 tsp cayenne pepper (0.5g)
- 1 tbsp (15g) peanut butter
- 1 clove garlic, minced
- 1/2 tsp (2.5g) grated ginger

Directions:

1. Cut the chicken breasts into bite-sized pieces.

2. In a small bowl, combine the light coconut milk, brown sugar, low-sodium soy sauce, ground cumin, ground coriander, turmeric, and cayenne pepper.

3. Stir to mix well.

4. In another small bowl, mix together the minced garlic, grated ginger, and peanut butter.

5. Place the chicken pieces in a bowl. Pour the coconut milk mixture over the chicken, tossing to ensure the chicken is evenly coated.

6. Thread the marinated chicken pieces onto skewers.

7. Preheat a grill or grill pan to medium-high heat.

8. Grill the chicken skewers for about 5-7 minutes on each side, or until the chicken is cooked through.

9. Serve the grilled chicken satay with the peanut sauce on the side.

Nutrition: Calories: 233.5; Fat: 9g; Carbs: 13g; Protein: 24g

Easy Fried Eggplant

Preparation time: 20 minutes   Cooking time: 15 minutes

Ingredients:

- 1/2 large eggplant, sliced into rounds
- Salt to sweat eggplant
- 1/2 cup (60g) whole wheat flour
- 1 egg, lightly beaten
- 1/2 cup (60g) whole wheat breadcrumbs
- Olive oil spray for frying

Directions:

1. Cut the eggplant into thin, uniform slices and sprinkle with salt. Let the eggplant sit for 30 minutes to allow it to sweat out some of its bitterness.

2. Rinse the salted eggplant slices and pat them dry with paper towels.

3. Prepare a breading station with three shallow bowls: one for the whole wheat flour, one for the lightly beaten egg, and one for the whole wheat breadcrumbs.

4. Dip each eggplant slice first in flour, then in the beaten egg, and finally coat them with breadcrumbs. Press the breadcrumbs onto the slices to help them adhere.

5. Heat olive oil in a skillet over medium-high heat. Use olive oil spray to coat the pan. Once the oil is hot, add the breaded eggplant slices to the skillet. Cook for 3-4 minutes on each side or until golden brown and crispy.

6. Remove the fried eggplant slices from the skillet using a slotted spoon. Place them on a plate lined with paper towels to drain excess oil. Serve the fried eggplant warm.

Nutrition: Calories: 358.5; Fat: 7g; Carbs: 60.5g; Protein: 13g

Simple Lemon-Herb Chicken

Preparation time: 5 minutes   Cooking time: 10 minutes

Ingredients:

- 2 boneless chicken breasts (200g each)
- 2 tbsp (30ml) fresh lemon juice
- 1 clove garlic, minced
- 1/2 tsp dried thyme (0.9g)
- Salt and pepper, to taste

- 2 tbsp (30g) whole wheat flour
- 1 tbsp (15ml) olive oil
- 2 tbsp (30ml) low-sodium chicken broth
- 1/2 tsp dried basil (0.9g)
- 2 tbsp chopped fresh parsley (6g)

Directions:

1. Season the chicken breasts with salt and pepper, then coat them in whole wheat flour.
2. Heat olive oil in a large skillet over medium-high heat.
3. Once the oil is hot, add the chicken breasts. Fry them for 4-5 minutes on each side, or until they are golden brown and cooked through.
4. Remove the chicken from the skillet and set it aside.
5. In the same skillet, add the low-sodium chicken broth, lemon juice, minced garlic, dried thyme, and dried basil.
6. Bring the mixture to a boil.
7. Boil for 2 to 3 minutes, or until the sauce has thickened slightly.
8. Return the chicken to the skillet, spooning some of the sauce over the chicken.
9. Cook the chicken for an additional 2 to 3 minutes, or until it is thoroughly heated and the flavors are well combined.
10. Garnish with chopped fresh parsley before serving.

Nutrition: Calories: 211; Fat: 9g; Carbs: 4g; Protein: 29.5g

Rustic Vegetable and Bean Soup

Preparation time: 10 minutes   Cooking time: 15 minutes

Ingredients:

- 1/2 tbsp (7.5ml) olive oil
- 1/4 cup (30g) chopped celery
- 1/4 cup (30g) chopped shallots
- 1 clove garlic, minced
- 1/2 tbsp chopped fresh marjoram
- 1/4 cup (30g) chopped carrots
- 1/4 cup (75g) diced gold potatoes
- 1/4 cup (30g) chopped tomatoes
- 1 ½ cups (360ml) low-sodium vegetable broth
- 1/2 can navy beans, drained and rinsed (210g)
- 1 tsp red wine vinegar (5ml)
- 2 tbsp (4g) thinly sliced chives

Directions:

1. Heat the olive oil in a 4-quart soup pot over medium heat.
2. Add the chopped celery and shallots to the pot.
3. Season with salt and black pepper.
4. Stir the vegetables occasionally until they start to soften.
5. Stir in the minced garlic and fresh marjoram and cook for an additional minute until fragrant.
6. Add the chopped carrots, diced potatoes, and chopped tomatoes to the pot.
7. Stir to mix them with the seasonings and aromatics.
8. Pour in the vegetable broth and bring the mixture to a boil.
9. Partially cover the pot and simmer until the vegetables are nearly tender, usually for about 10 to 20 minutes.
10. Stir in the navy beans and any reserved tomato juices. Add the rest of the broth.
11. Continue to simmer the soup with a partial cover for about 10 more minutes to allow the flavors to meld.
12. Ladle the soup into serving bowls. Garnish each bowl with thinly sliced chives.
13. Serve the soup warm.

Nutrition: Calories: 236 Fat: 5g; Carbs: 34.5g; Protein: 14g

Easy Chorizo Street Tacos

Preparation time: 10 minutes   Cooking time: 10 minutes

Ingredients:

- 1/2 pound lean turkey chorizo (230g)
- 1/4 cup (30g) diced onion
- 1/4 cup (30g) diced bell pepper
- Salt and pepper, to taste
- 4 small corn tortillas
- Toppings: cilantro, diced onion, diced tomatoes, low-fat sour cream, lime wedges

Directions:

1. In a large skillet over medium-high heat, cook the chorizo for 5-7 minutes, stirring occasionally, until it is browned.
2. Add the diced bell pepper and onion to the skillet. Continue cooking for about 5 minutes, or until the vegetables are softened.
3. Season the chorizo mixture with salt and pepper to taste.
4. In a separate skillet, warm the corn tortillas over medium heat until they are warm and slightly charred.
5. To assemble the tacos, place a few spoonfuls of the chorizo mixture onto each tortilla. Top with cilantro, additional diced onion, diced tomatoes, a dollop of low-fat sour cream, and a squeeze of lime juice.
6. Serve the tacos warm.

Nutrition: Calories: 131; Fat: 6.5g; Carbs: 13g; Protein: 5g

Moroccan Spiced Red Lentils Stew

Preparation time: 15 minutes   Cooking time: 50 minutes

Ingredients:

- 1 1/2 cups (360ml) low-sodium vegetable broth
- 1/6 cup (30g) dry millet
- 1/4 tbsp (3.75ml) olive oil
- 1 tbsp (15g) tomato paste
- Pinch of cayenne pepper
- 1/2 cup (100g) dried lentils, rinsed
- 1/4 cup (30g) finely sliced onion
- 1/4 cup (30g) finely sliced red bell pepper
- 1/2 celery stalk, sliced

- Pinch of ground cinnamon
- 1/4 cup (30g) sliced dried apricots
- 1/2 tbsp (3.75g) ground coriander
- 1/4 tbsp (1.25g) ground cumin

Directions:

1. Heat the olive oil in a 3-quart stockpot or skillet over medium heat.
2. Add the onion and cook for about 6 minutes, stirring frequently, until it becomes fragrant and translucent.
3. Stir in the millet, lentils, and vegetable broth. Bring the mixture to a boil.
4. Add the dried apricots, cayenne pepper, ground coriander, ground cumin, tomato paste, sliced bell pepper, sliced celery, and salt to taste.
5. Reduce the heat, cover the pot, and simmer for 35 to 45 minutes, or until the lentils and millet are tender. Serve the stew hot.

Nutrition: Calories: 286.5; Fat: 3.5g; Carbs: 48g; Protein: 16.5g

Garlic Ranch Chicken

Preparation time: 10 minutes   Cooking time: 20 minutes

Ingredients:

- 2 boneless chicken breasts (200g each)
- 1/4 cup (60ml) low-fat buttermilk
- 1/2 tsp (2.5ml) dried chives
- 1/2 tsp (2.5ml) onion powder
- 1/4 tsp salt (1.50g)
- 1/8 tsp black pepper (0.30g)
- 2 tbsp (30g) whole wheat flour
- 1/8 cup (30g) low-fat mayonnaise
- 1 clove garlic, minced
- 1 tbsp (15ml) chopped fresh dill
- 2 tbsp (30ml) olive oil

Directions:

1. In a large bowl, combine the low-fat buttermilk, parsley (not listed in ingredients but likely intended), low-fat mayonnaise, minced garlic, onion powder, chopped dill, dried chives, salt, and pepper to make the marinade.

2. Add the chicken breasts to the bowl, ensuring they are well coated with the marinade. For optimal flavor, cover and refrigerate for at least an hour or overnight.

3. Place the whole wheat flour in a shallow dish.

4. Remove the chicken from the marinade, allowing any excess to drip off. Dredge the chicken in the flour to coat evenly.

5. Heat olive oil in a large pan over medium heat.

6. Once the oil is hot, add the chicken breasts. Cook for about 8 minutes per side, or until they are golden brown and cooked through.

7. Remove the chicken from the pan and place on a plate lined with paper towels to absorb any excess oil.

8. Serve the Garlic Ranch Chicken with your choice of sides, such as roasted vegetables, mashed potatoes, or a salad.

Nutrition: Calories: 132; Fat: 6g; Carbs: 3.5g; Protein: 15g

Flounder Tacos with Cabbage Slaw

Preparation time: 10 minutes   Cooking time: 6 minutes

Ingredients:

- 1 tbsp (15ml) freshly squeezed lime juice
- 1/2 cup (35g) thinly sliced red cabbage
- 1/4 avocado, chopped
- 1 ½ tbsp (22.5ml) olive oil, divided

- 1/2 tbsp (7.5g) ground cumin
- 4 ounces (115g) skinless flounder fillets, sliced into 1-inch chunks
- 2 corn tortillas, warmed
- Pinch of salt and pepper
- Fresh cilantro, for garnish

Directions:

1. In a small bowl, combine the ground cumin, a pinch of salt, and pepper with the flounder chunks. Toss to coat the fish evenly.

2. In another small bowl, mix together the thinly sliced red cabbage, chopped avocado, 1 teaspoon of olive oil, and freshly squeezed lime juice.

3. Heat the remaining 2 teaspoons of olive oil in a medium-sized pan over medium-high heat.

4. Add the seasoned flounder to the skillet. Cook for about 4 minutes, turning occasionally, until the fish is nearly opaque and flakes easily with a fork.

5. Divide the flounder among two warm corn tortillas. Top each tortilla with the cabbage avocado slaw. Garnish the tacos with fresh cilantro and serve.

Nutrition: Calories: 206.5; Fat: 10g; Carbs: 14g; Protein: 16g

Easy Baked Tilapia

Preparation time: 5 minutes   Cooking time: 25 minutes

Ingredients:

- 2 Tilapia fillets (100g each)
- Salt and pepper, to taste
- 1 tbsp (15ml) olive oil

- 1 clove garlic, minced
- 1 tbsp (15ml) lemon juice
- 2 tbsp (8g) chopped fresh parsley

Directions:

1. Preheat the oven to 375°F (190°C). Season the Tilapia fillets with salt and pepper.

2. In a small bowl, mix together the olive oil, chopped parsley, lemon juice, and minced garlic.

3. Place the Tilapia fillets in a baking dish. Brush the olive oil mixture over the fish, ensuring they are well coated.

4. Bake in the preheated oven for 10 to 15 minutes, or until the Tilapia is cooked through and flakes easily with a fork.

5. Serve the baked Tilapia with your choice of sides, such as roasted vegetables, rice, or a fresh salad.

Nutrition: Calories: 86; Fat: 2g; Carbs: 3.5g; Protein: 12.5g

Tuna Fish Pea Salad

Preparation time: 5 minutes   Cooking time: 10 minutes

Ingredients:

- 1/2 can of tuna fish, drained (about 50g)
- 1/2 cup (about 70g) of thawed frozen peas
- 2 tbsp (about 15g) minced onion
- 2 tbsp (30g) low-fat mayonnaise
- 1/2 tbsp (7.5ml) lemon juice
- Salt and pepper, to taste

Directions:

1. In a large bowl, combine the drained tuna fish, thawed peas, and minced onion.
2. In a separate small bowl, mix together the low-fat mayonnaise, lemon juice, and a pinch of salt and pepper.
3. Pour the mayonnaise mixture over the tuna and pea mixture in the large bowl.
4. Gently toss the salad to ensure all ingredients are evenly coated with the mayonnaise dressing.
5. Cover the bowl and refrigerate for at least 30 minutes to allow the flavors to meld together.
6. Serve the Tuna Fish Pea Salad on a bed of lettuce or use it as a filling for a sandwich.

Nutrition: Calories: 51.5; Fat: 0.5g; Carbs: 3.5g; Protein: 8.5g

Loaded Sweet Potatoes

Preparation time: 5 minutes

Cooking time: 80 minutes

Ingredients:

- 1 medium sweet potato (100g each half)
- 1/4 avocado, sliced
- 1/6 cup (55ml) water
- 1/2 garlic clove, minced
- 1/2 can black beans, drained (100g)
- Salt and pepper, to taste
- 2 cups (134g) chopped kale leaves
- 1/4 cup (35g) halved grape tomatoes

Directions:

1. Preheat the oven to 375°F (190°C) and line a baking pan with parchment paper.
2. Prick the sweet potatoes several times with a fork. Bake them for 45 to 60 minutes, or until they are soft.
3. Meanwhile, heat a medium-sized pot over medium heat. Sauté the minced garlic for about 1 minute, or until fragrant.
4. Add the kale and grape tomatoes to the pot. Pour in the water and cover. Cook for 5 minutes.
5. Continue cooking the vegetables, uncovered, for an additional 15 minutes, stirring occasionally, until they are tender but still bright green.
6. Stir in the black beans and heat through. Season with salt and pepper to taste.
7. Split the baked sweet potatoes lengthwise into two halves.
8. Top each sweet potato half with the black bean and kale mixture, and sliced avocado.
9. Serve the Loaded Sweet Potatoes hot.

Nutrition: Calories: 375.5; Fat: 7.5g; Carbs: 66.5g; Protein: 14g

Creamy Quinoa, Lentils, and Vegetables

Preparation time: 15 minutes   Cooking time: 45 minutes

Ingredients:

For the lentils

- 1/8 cup (25g) dried black lentils
- 1/4 cup (60ml) water

- Pinch salt

For the roasted carrots and beets

- 1/4 pound (60g) rainbow carrots with stems

- Olive oil nonstick cooking spray
- 1 medium beet, peeled and sliced

For the creamy quinoa

- 3/8 cup (90ml) low-sodium vegetable broth
- 3/8 cup (90ml) unsweetened almond milk, divided
- 1/4 cup (45g) quinoa, rinsed
- 1/4 teaspoon onion powder
- 1/8 teaspoon garlic powder
- 1/2 cup (33g) chopped Swiss chard
- 1/2 tbsp (4g) chopped fresh parsley

Directions:

1. To make the lentils

In a saucepan over medium heat, set together the lentils, water, and salt and set to a boil. Seal, lower the heat to medium-low, and simmer for 35 to 40 minutes.

To make the roasted carrots and beets

1. Set the oven temperature to 400°F and prepare the baking sheet by lining it with a sheet of parchment paper.
2. Wash the carrots well and remove extra roots and leaves, leaving roughly 2 inches of stem.
3. Lightly spray the lined baking sheet with cooking spray, add the carrots and beets, then spray them lightly with cooking spray.
4. Whisk with salt and pepper to season. Toast for 25 to 30 minutes, or until the vegetables are fork-tender and beginning to brown.

To make the creamy quinoa

1. In a large, partly covered pan over medium heat, combine the vegetable broth, 1/4 cup of almond milk, quinoa, onion powder, and garlic powder.
2. Set the heat to medium, bring to a boil, and then simmer the quinoa for 15 to 20 minutes, or until it is tender.
3. Continue cooking and stirring while adding the final 1/4 cup of almond milk.
4. When all the milk is added and the quinoa has a light creaminess to it, add the cooked lentils, chard, and parsley.
5. Set off the heat and stir until the chard is slightly wilted.
6. Add salt and pepper.
7. Divide between two bowls, top with the roasted vegetables and almonds, garnish with parsley, and serve.

Nutrition: Calories: 222.5; Fat: 5.5g; Carbs: 35g; Protein: 10

Shrimp and Rice Noodle Salad

Preparation time: 15 minutes   Cooking time: 5 minutes

Ingredients:

- 4 oz (115g) rice noodles
- 1/2 lb (230g) large shrimp, peeled and deveined
- 1 clove garlic, sliced
- 1 tbsp (15ml) fish sauce
- 1 tbsp (15ml) rice vinegar
- 1 tbsp (15g) brown sugar
- 1/2 tbsp (7.5ml) low-sodium soy sauce

- 1/8 tsp red pepper flakes
- 2 tbsp (8g) sliced fresh cilantro
- 2 tbsp (8g) minced fresh mint
- 2 tbsp (8g) sliced fresh basil
- 2 tbsp (about 15g) minced peanuts
- 2 tbsp (about 15g) sliced green onions
- Lime slices for serving

Directions:

1. Prepare the rice noodles according to the instructions on the package.
2. Heat a small amount of oil in a large skillet over medium-high heat.
3. Add the shrimp and garlic to the skillet. Sauté for 2 to 3 minutes on each side, until the shrimp are pink and fully cooked.
4. In a small bowl, combine the fish sauce, rice vinegar, brown sugar, low-sodium soy sauce, and red pepper flakes.
5. In a large bowl, arrange the cooked rice noodles, cooked shrimp, fresh basil, mint, cilantro, minced peanuts, and sliced green onions.
6. Drizzle the dressing over the salad and toss everything together to combine.
7. Serve the salad garnished with lime slices.

Nutrition: Calories: 136.5; Fat: 3g; Carbs: 18.45g; Protein: 8.4

SALAD RECIPES

Roasted New Red Potatoes

Preparation time: 5 minutes   Cooking time: 20 minutes

Ingredients:

- 1/2 lb (225g) new red potatoes, washed and dried
- 1 tbsp (15ml) olive oil
- 1/2 tsp dried thyme
- Salt and pepper, to taste

Directions:

1. Preheat the oven to 425°F (220°C).
2. Cut the new red potatoes into wedges, about 1/2 inch thick.
3. In a large bowl, toss the potato wedges with olive oil, dried thyme, and a pinch of salt and pepper until they are evenly coated.
4. Arrange the potatoes on a baking sheet in a single layer.
5. Roast in the oven for 20-25 minutes, or until the potatoes are tender and golden brown. Remember to flip the potatoes halfway through the cooking time to ensure even browning.

Nutrition: Calories: 84.5; Fat: 3.5g; Carbs: 13.5g; Protein: 1.5g

Potato Dumplings

Preparation time: 20 minutes   Cooking time: 45 minutes

Ingredients:

- 2 cups (500g) mashed potatoes
- 1/4 cup (30g) all-purpose flour
- 1/2 egg, beaten
- 2 tbsp (15g) grated onion
- 1 clove garlic, minced
- 1/2 tsp salt
- 1/8 tsp black pepper
- 2 tbsp (7.5g) chopped fresh parsley
- Flour for dusting
- Water or low-sodium chicken broth for boiling

Directions:

1. In a large mixing bowl, combine the mashed potatoes, grated onion, 1/4 cup all-purpose flour, beaten half egg, minced garlic, salt, pepper, and chopped parsley. Mix thoroughly.
2. Form the mixture into 1½ -inch balls. Lightly dust them with extra flour.
3. Bring a large saucepan of water or chicken broth to a simmer.
4. Gently drop the dumplings into the simmering water or broth. Be careful not to overcrowd the pot.
5. Cook the dumplings until they float to the top, about 8 to 10 minutes.
6. Use a slotted spoon to remove the dumplings from the water and place them on a plate lined with paper towels to drain any excess water.
7. Optionally, you can fry the dumplings in a pan for a crispy exterior.

Nutrition: Calories: 138.5; Fat: 5g; Carbs: 21g; Protein: 3g

Marinated Carrot Salad

Preparation time: 20 minutes   Cooking time: 10 minutes

Ingredients:

- 2 cups (240g) thinly sliced carrots
- 1/4 cup (60ml) white wine vinegar
- 2 tbsp (30ml) olive oil
- 1 clove garlic, minced

- 1/2 tsp honey
- 1/2 tsp Dijon mustard
- Salt and pepper, to taste
- Fresh parsley or cilantro, chopped (optional)

Directions:

1. Place the thinly sliced carrots in a bowl.
2. In a separate bowl, whisk together the white wine vinegar, olive oil, minced garlic, honey, Dijon mustard, and a pinch of salt and pepper.
3. Drizzle the marinade over the sliced carrots and toss well to ensure the carrots are evenly coated.

4. Cover the bowl and refrigerate for at least two hours to allow the carrots to marinate and absorb the flavors. Before serving, remove the salad from the refrigerator and let it sit for about 15 minutes to come to room temperature.

5. Optionally, garnish the salad with chopped fresh parsley or cilantro.

6. Serve the marinated carrot salad either chilled or at room temperature.

Nutrition: Calories: 83; Fat: 4g; Carbs: 12g; Protein: 1g

Tofu Salad

Preparation time: 15 minutes　　　　　　　Cooking time: 30 minutes

Ingredients:

- Half Block of firm tofu, cubed (200g)
- 2 tbsp red bell pepper, sliced (30g)
- 2 tbsp cucumber, minced (30g)
- 2 tbsp red onion, chopped (30g)
- 1 tbsp rice vinegar (15ml)
- 1 tbsp low-sodium soy sauce (15ml)

- 1/2 tbsp sesame oil (7.5ml)
- 1/2 tsp grated ginger (2.5ml)
- 1/2 clove of garlic, mashed
- Salt and pepper, to taste
- Garnishes: sesame seeds and chopped green onions (optional)

Directions:

1. Drain and press the tofu to remove any excess water. Then cube the tofu.

2. In a large bowl, combine the cubed tofu, sliced red bell pepper, minced cucumber, and chopped red onion.

3. In a small bowl, whisk together the rice vinegar, soy sauce, sesame oil, grated ginger, mashed garlic, and a pinch of salt and pepper.

4. Pour the dressing over the tofu mixture and toss to ensure everything is well combined.

5. Cover the bowl and refrigerate for at least 30 minutes to allow the flavors to meld.

6. Before serving, remove the salad from the refrigerator and let it sit for about 15 minutes to come to room temperature.

7. Optionally, garnish the salad with sesame seeds and chopped green onions.

8. Serve the Tofu Salad chilled or at room temperature.

Nutrition: Calories: 72.5; Fat: 4.5g; Carbs: 5g; Protein: 4g

Tomato Cucumber Salad

Preparation time: 10 minutes

Cooking time: 5 minutes

Ingredients:

- 1 cup diced tomatoes (150g)
- 1/2 cup diced cucumber (75g)
- 2 tbsp red onion, diced (30g)
- 1 tbsp red wine vinegar (15ml)
- 1/2 tbsp olive oil (7.5ml)

- 1/2 tsp honey (2.5ml)
- 1/2 clove garlic, minced
- Salt and pepper, to taste
- Fresh basil or parsley, chopped (optional)

Directions:

1. In a bowl, combine the diced tomatoes, cucumber, and red onion.
2. In a small bowl, whisk together the red wine vinegar, olive oil, honey, minced garlic, and a pinch of salt and pepper to create the dressing.
3. Pour the dressing over the tomato, cucumber, and onion mixture. Toss everything together to ensure the vegetables are well coated.
4. Cover the bowl and refrigerate for at least 30 minutes, allowing the flavors to meld.
5. Before serving, remove the salad from the refrigerator and let it sit for about 15 minutes to come to room temperature.
6. Optionally, garnish the salad with chopped fresh basil or parsley.
7. Serve the Tomato Cucumber Salad chilled or at room temperature.

Nutrition: Calories: 52; Fat: 4g; Carbs: 3.5g; Protein: 1g

Quinoa Spinach Power Salad

Preparation time: 5 minutes

Cooking time: 10 minutes

Ingredients:

- 1 cup spinach, finely sliced (30g)
- 1/2 cup sugar snap peas (60g)

- 3/4 tbsp olive oil (11ml)
- 1/8 tsp salt

- 1/2 cup diced tomato (75g)
- 3/4 tbsp lemon juice (11ml)
- 1/4 cup diced cucumber (30g)
- 2 tbsp sliced almonds (15g)

- 1 cup water (240ml)
- 1/4 cup uncooked quinoa, rinsed (45g)
- 1/8 tsp black pepper

Directions:

1. In a medium pot, bring the water to a boil.
2. Add the quinoa and continue boiling for 10 minutes or until the quinoa is tender.
3. Drain the quinoa and allow it to cool.
4. In a large bowl, combine the sliced spinach, sugar snap peas, diced tomato, diced cucumber, sliced almonds, and cooled quinoa.
5. In a small bowl, whisk together the lemon juice, olive oil, salt, and black pepper.
6. Pour the dressing over the salad and toss to ensure the ingredients are well coated.
7. Divide the salad between two serving bowls and enjoy.

Nutrition: Calories: 161; Fat: 9g; Carbs: 16g; Protein: 5.5g

Salad of Kale, Avocado, and Carrots

Preparation time: 10 minutes   Cooking time: 30 minutes

Ingredients:

- 2 cups kale, stemmed and chopped (134g)
- 1/4 can chickpeas, drained and rinsed (100g)
- 1/2 large avocado, cubed (100g)
- 1 tbsp walnuts, chopped (7.5g)

- 1/2 cup baby carrots, halved lengthwise (60g)
- 1/2 tbsp olive oil (7.5ml)
- 1 tbsp lemon juice (15ml)
- Salt and pepper, to taste

Directions:

1. Preheat the oven to 400°F (205°C).
2. In a small bowl, toss the baby carrots with olive oil, and a pinch of salt and pepper.

3. Spread the seasoned carrots on a rimmed baking sheet and roast for 20 minutes in the preheated oven.

4. Add the chickpeas and chopped walnuts to the baking sheet with the carrots.

5. Return to the oven and continue to bake for an additional 5 to 10 minutes, or until the carrots are tender and golden.

6. Massage the kale with your hands for about two minutes until it softens and turns a brighter green.

7. In a large serving bowl, combine the massaged kale with lemon juice and half of the cubed avocado. Add half of the roasted carrot, chickpea, and walnut mixture to the bowl with the kale and toss well.

8. Top the salad with the remaining avocado and the rest of the roasted carrot mixture. Divide the salad between two serving dishes and enjoy.

Nutrition: Calories: 267.5; Fat: 15g; Carbs: 29g; Protein: 8.5g

Fruit Punch Salad

Preparation time: 10 minutes

Cooking time: 5 minutes

Ingredients:

- 1/2 can fruit cocktail, drained (200g)
- 1/2 can pineapple chunks, drained (200g)
- 1/2 banana, sliced (60g)
- 1/2 cup mini marshmallows (30g)
- 1/4 cup shredded coconut (20g)
- 1/4 cup low-fat sour cream (60ml)
- 2 tbsp sugar (25g)
- 2 tbsp orange juice (30ml)
- 1/2 tbsp lemon juice (7.5ml)

Directions:

1. In a large bowl, combine the fruit cocktail, pineapple chunks, sliced banana, mini marshmallows, and shredded coconut.

2. In a separate small bowl, mix together the low-fat sour cream, sugar, orange juice, and lemon juice to make the dressing.

3. Pour the sour cream mixture over the fruit mixture and stir until everything is well combined.

4. Cover the bowl and refrigerate for at least 2 hours to allow the flavors to meld.

5. Before serving, remove the salad from the refrigerator and let it sit for about 15 minutes to come to room temperature. Serve chilled.

6. Optionally, you can add other fruits like strawberries, blueberries, or any berries of your choice to enhance the salad.

Nutrition: Calories: 135; Fat: 0g; Carbs: 34g; Protein: 2g

Avocado and Eggs Salad

Preparation time: 5 minutes

Cooking time: 10 minutes

Ingredients:

- 2 large eggs
- Salt and pepper, to taste
- 1/2 tbsp butter or oil (7.5ml)
- 2 cups mixed greens (60g)
- 1/2 avocado, diced (100g)
- 1/8 cup cherry tomatoes, halved (15g)
- 1/8 cup red onion, thinly sliced (15g)
- 1 tbsp balsamic vinegar (15ml)
- 1/2 tbsp olive oil (7.5ml)
- 1/2 tsp honey (2.5ml)
- 1/2 clove garlic, minced
- 1/8 tsp Dijon mustard

Directions:

1. Bring a pot of water to a boil in a saucepan. Use a slotted spoon to carefully lower the eggs into the water.

2. For soft-boiled eggs, cook for 6–8 minutes; for hard-boiled eggs, cook for 10–12 minutes. Remove the eggs from the water and place them in an ice bath to cool.

3. Heat the butter or oil in a skillet over medium heat.

4. Add the mixed greens to the skillet and cook for 1-2 minutes, just until they begin to wilt.

5. In a small bowl, whisk together balsamic vinegar, olive oil, honey, minced garlic, and Dijon mustard.

6. In a large bowl, combine the cooked greens, diced avocado, halved cherry tomatoes, and thinly sliced red onion.

7. Drizzle the dressing over the salad and toss gently to combine.

8. Peel the cooled eggs and cut them into wedges.

9. Place the egg wedges on top of the salad.

10. Season with salt and pepper to taste.

Nutrition: Calories: 88; Fat: 6.5g; Carbs: 4g; Protein: 4.5g

Gingered Beef and Broccoli Salad Bowl

Preparation time: 20 minutes   Cooking time: 10 minutes

Ingredients:

- 1/2 pound flank steak (225g)
- 2 tbsp soy sauce (30ml)
- 1 tbsp rice vinegar (15ml)
- 1 tbsp brown sugar (12.5g)
- 1 tbsp grated ginger (15ml)
- 1 clove garlic, minced
- 1 tbsp cornstarch (7.5g)
- 1 tbsp vegetable oil (15ml)
- 2 cups broccoli florets (150g)
- 1 cup cooked brown rice (150g)

Directions:

1. In a large bowl, combine the rice vinegar, soy sauce, brown sugar, ginger, and minced garlic to make the marinade.

2. Add the flank steak to the marinade, ensuring it is well coated.

3. Cover and refrigerate for at least 30 minutes to marinate.

4. In a shallow bowl, make a slurry by mixing the cornstarch with 2 tablespoons (30ml) of water.

5. Heat the vegetable oil in a large pan or wok over high heat.

6. Remove the steak from the marinade and add it to the hot pan.

7. Cook the steak for 2 to 3 minutes on each side, or until it's cooked to your preference. Remove the steak from the pan and let it rest for a few minutes before slicing it against the grain. In the same skillet, cook the broccoli florets until they are tender and slightly charred.

8. To assemble, divide the cooked brown rice among bowls.

9. Top with the sliced steak and broccoli.

Nutrition: Calories: 118.5; Fat: 4.5g; Carbs: 8.5g; Protein: 11g

Spinach, Pears, and Cranberries Salad

Preparation time: 15 minutes

Cooking time: 5 minutes

Ingredients:

- 3 cups fresh spinach leaves (90g)
- 1/8 cup red onion, sliced (15g)
- 1/8 cup crumbled blue cheese (15g)
- 1/8 cup dried cranberries (15g)

- 1 ripe pear, cored and diced (120g)
- 2 tbsp balsamic vinegar (30ml)
- 2 tbsp olive oil (30ml)
- 1/2 clove garlic, minced
- Salt and pepper, to taste

Directions:

1. In a large salad bowl, combine the spinach leaves, sliced red onion, crumbled blue cheese, dried cranberries, and diced pear.

2. In a small bowl, whisk together the balsamic vinegar, olive oil, minced garlic, and a pinch of salt and pepper to create the dressing.

3. Drizzle the dressing over the salad and toss gently to evenly coat the ingredients.

4. Allow the salad to sit for a few minutes before serving. Serve and enjoy the salad.

Nutrition: Calories: 107; Fat: 5.5g; Carbs: 12.5g; Protein: 2.5g

Zucchini Patties

Preparation time: 20 minutes

Cooking time: 10 minutes

Ingredients:

- 1 medium zucchini, grated (100g)

- 1/4 cup grated onion (30g)
- 1/4 cup all-purpose flour (30g)

- 1/4 cup grated Parmesan cheese (15g)
- 1 egg, beaten
- Salt and pepper, to taste
- 2 tbsp vegetable oil (30ml)

Directions:

1. In a large bowl, mix together the grated zucchini and onion.
2. Stir in the flour, grated Parmesan cheese, beaten egg, and a pinch of salt and pepper.
3. Combine everything well.
4. Heat the vegetable oil in a skillet over medium-high heat.
5. Using a spoon, scoop small portions of the zucchini mixture and form them into patties.
6. Gently place the patties in the hot skillet.
7. Cook them for 2-3 minutes on each side, or until they are golden brown and crispy.
8. Remove the patties from the skillet and place them on paper towels to drain any excess oil.
9. Serve the zucchini patties warm. They can be accompanied by your favorite dipping sauce.
10. Optional: Add herbs such as parsley, dill, or cilantro to the mixture for an added flavor boost.

Nutrition: Calories: 122.5; Fat: 7.5g; Carbs: 8g; Protein: 6.5g

Sweet and Spicy Tofu Salad with Carrot

Preparation time: 30 minutes

Cooking time: 20 minutes

Ingredients:

- 1/2 block firm tofu, cubed (200g)
- 1 tbsp soy sauce (15ml)
- 1/2 tbsp rice vinegar (7.5ml)
- 1/2 tbsp sesame oil (7.5ml)
- 1/2 tsp sriracha (2.5ml)
- 1 medium carrot, grated (60g)
- 1 green onion, thinly sliced
- 1/2 tbsp sesame seeds (optional) (7.5g)

Directions:

1. Cube the tofu and set it aside.

2. In a small bowl, whisk together the soy sauce, rice vinegar, sesame oil, and sriracha to create the dressing.

3. Heat a pan over medium-high heat. Once hot, add the tofu cubes and cook for 5 to 7 minutes, or until they are golden brown and crispy.

4. Remove the tofu from the pan and transfer it to a large bowl. Add the grated carrot, thinly sliced green onion, and sesame seeds (if using) to the bowl with the tofu.

5. Drizzle the dressing over the tofu and vegetables.

6. Toss everything together until well combined and evenly coated with the dressing.

7. Serve the salad immediately or refrigerate it before serving for a chilled salad option.

Nutrition: Calories: 300; Fat: 0g; Carbs: 43.5g; Protein: 14g

Marinated Cucumber & Tomato Salad

Preparation time: 15 minutes   Cooking time: 120 minutes

Ingredients:

- 1 large cucumber, skinned, halved, and thinly sliced (250g)
- 1 cup cherry tomatoes, halved (150g)
- 1/4 cup red onion, thinly sliced (30g)
- 1/8 cup chopped fresh parsley (15g)

- 2 tbsp white wine vinegar (30ml)
- 1 tbsp olive oil (15ml)
- 1/2 tbsp honey (7.5ml)
- 1/2 tsp Dijon mustard (2.5ml)
- 1/4 tsp salt
- 1/8 tsp black pepper

Directions:

1. In a large bowl, mix the sliced cucumbers, halved cherry tomatoes, thinly sliced red onion, and chopped parsley.

2. In a small bowl, whisk together the white wine vinegar, olive oil, honey, Dijon mustard, salt, and black pepper to make the dressing.

3. Pour the dressing over the cucumber and tomato mixture. Toss gently to ensure all the ingredients are well coated with the dressing.

4. Cover the salad and refrigerate for at least 2 hours, or up to 8 hours, to allow the flavors to meld together. This marination time is crucial for developing the flavors.

5. Before serving, give the salad a good toss to redistribute the dressing and flavors.

Nutrition: Calories: 45; Fat: 3.5g; Carbs: 3g; Protein: 0.5g

Wilted Spinach and Tilapia Salad

Preparation time: 20 minutes   Cooking time: 5 minutes

Ingredients:

- 2 tilapia fillets (200g each)
- Salt and pepper, to taste
- 1 tbsp olive oil (15ml)
- 2 cups fresh spinach leaves (60g)
- 1/8 cup red onion, thinly sliced (15g)
- 1/8 cup cherry tomatoes, halved (15g)
- 1 tbsp lemon juice (15ml)
- 1/2 tbsp balsamic vinegar (7.5ml)
- 1/2 tbsp honey (7.5ml)
- 1/2 clove garlic, minced
- 1/8 tsp Dijon mustard

Directions:

1. In a large bowl, mix the sliced cucumbers, halved cherry tomatoes, thinly sliced red onion, and chopped parsley.

2. In a small bowl, whisk together the white wine vinegar, olive oil, honey, Dijon mustard, salt, and black pepper to make the dressing.

3. Pour the dressing over the cucumber and tomato mixture.

4. Toss gently to ensure all the ingredients are well coated with the dressing.

5. Cover the salad and refrigerate for at least 2 hours, or up to 8 hours, to allow the flavors to meld together. Before serving, give the salad a good toss to redistribute the dressing and flavors.

Nutrition: Calories: 93; Fat: 4.5g; Carbs: 4g; Protein: 10g

30-DAY MEAL PLAN

DAY	BREAKFAST	LUNCH	DINNER	SALAD
1	Peanut Butter Banana Outmeal	Turkey and Spinach Rice Bowl	Pocket Eggs with Sesame Sauce	Marinated Cucumber & Tomato Salad
	pg.15	*pg.32*	*pg.68*	*pg.120*
2	Muesli with Raspberries	Pesto Pasta	Lentil Walnut Burgers	Avocado and Eggs Salad
	pg.25	*pg.59*	*pg.69*	*pg.116*
3	Pistachio & Peach Toast	Shrimp Scampi with Zoodles	Lemon-Thyme Chicken	Salad of Kale, Avocado, and Carrots
	pg.22	*pg.53*	*pg.92*	*pg.114*
4	Spinach Omelet	Rainbow Trout Baked in Foil	Broccoli and Gold Potato Soup	Fruit Punch Salad
	pg.12	*pg.50*	*pg.87*	*pg.115*
5	Bagel Avocado Toast	Broiled Tuna Steaks with Lime	Cauliflower Fried Rice	Spinach, Pears and Cranberries Salad
	pg.20	*pg.55*	*pg.81*	*pg.118*
6	Carrot Baked Oatmeal	Bourbon Steak	Mushroom Frittata	Zucchini Patties
	pg.19	*pg.39*	*pg.76*	*pg.118*
7	Shrimp salad with avocado	Maple Salmon	Zucchini "Spaghetti" with Almond Pesto	Tofu Salad
	pg.14	*pg.41*	*pg.70*	*pg.112*
8	Lentil Asparagus Omelet	Green Beans and Mushrooms Spaghetti	Chicken Kebabs	Potato Dumplings
	pg.13	*pg.47*	*pg.65*	*pg.110*

9	Breakfast Parfait	Sesame-Crusted Tuna Steaks	Acorn Squash Stuffed with White Beans	Sweet and Spicy Tofu Salad with Carrots
	pg.24	*pg.51*	*pg.89*	*pg.119*
10	Healthy Bread Pudding	Easy Keto Korean Beef with Cauli Rice	Portobello Mushroom with Mozzarella	Fruit Punch Salad
	pg.25	*pg.36*	*pg.64*	*pg.115*
11	Cannellini Bean & Herbed Ricotta Toast	Turkey Sandwich	Indian Spiced Cauliflower Fried Rice	Wilted Spinach and Tilapia Salad
	pg.26	*pg.49*	*pg.66*	*pg.121*
12	Summer Berry Parfait with Yogurt	Black Bean Risotto	Seared Tilapia with Spiralized Zucchini	Tofu Salad
	pg.29	*pg.45*	*pg.86*	*pg.112*
13	Egg Tartine	Chicken Kebabs Mexicana	Salmon with Creamy Feta Cucumbers	Roasted New Red Potatoes
	pg.27	*pg.60*	*pg.82*	*pg.110*
14	Strawberry Peach Smoothie	Lemon Garlic Mackerel	Spring Minestrone Soup	Fruit Punch Salad
	pg.23	*pg.54*	*pg.91*	*pg.115*
15	Peanut Butter Banana Oatmeal	Two-Mushroom Barley Soup	Chicken Satay	Roasted New Red Potatoes
	pg.15	*pg.33*	*pg.97*	*pg.110*
16	Raspberry Mousse	Fish Chowder Sheet Pan Bake	Grilled Squash Garlic Bread	Avocado and Eggs Salad
	pg.29	*pg.40*	*pg.78*	*pg.116*
17	Tofu Scramble	Chopped Power Salad with Chicken	Braised Cauliflower and Squash Penne	Creamy Quinoa, Lentils, and Vegetables
	pg.28	*pg.43*	*pg.75*	*pg.106*

18	Southwestern Waffle	Chicken Cutlets with Pineapple Rice	Tarragon Sweet Potato and Egg Skillet	Tomato Cucumber Salad
	pg.21	*pg.61*	*pg.73*	*pg.113*
19	Pineapple Grapefruit Detox Smoothie	Spaghetti Squash and Chickpea Sauté	Farro with Sun-Dried Tomatoes	Spinach, Pears, and Cranberries Salad
	pg.21	*pg.57*	*pg.71*	*pg.118*
20	Spinach & Egg Scramble with Raspberries	Maple Salmon	Tofu Vegetable Stir-Fry	Quinoa Spinach Power Salad
	pg.19	*pg.41*	*pg.67*	*pg.113*
21	Shrimp Salad with Avocado	Easy Keto Korean Beef with Cauli Rice	Salmon with Creamy Feta Cucumbers	Zucchini Patties Creamy
	pg.14	*pg.36*	*pg.82*	*pg.118*
22	Muesli with Raspberries	Fried Chicken Bowl	Creamy Chicken and Chickpea Salad	Loaded Sweet Potatoes
	pg.25	*pg.35*	*pg.86*	*pg.105*
23	Cannellini Bean & Herbed Ricotta Toast	Salmon and Summer Squash in Parchment	Simple Tomato Soup	Marinated Carrots Salad
	pg.26	*pg.49*	*pg.85*	*pg.111*
24	Bagel Avocado Toasts	Turkey and Spinach Rice Bowl	Lemon-Thyme Chicken	Tofu Salad
	pg.20	*pg.32*	*pg.92*	*pg.112*
25	Summer Berry Parfait with Yogurt	Chicken and Pesto Sourdough Sandwich	Mushroom Frittata	Potato Dumplings
	pg.29	*pg.32*	*pg.76*	*pg.110*
26	Coconut Milk Pudding	Pan-Seared Pork and Fried Tomato Salad	One Skillet Quinoa and Vegetable	Gingered Beef and Broccoli Salad Bowl
	pg.17	*pg.38*	*pg.72*	*pg.117*

27	Almond Butter & Roasted Grape Toast	Hawaiian Chop Steaks	Pocket Eggs with Sesame Sauce	Sweet and Spicy Tofu Salad with Carrot
	pg.24	*pg.41*	*pg.68*	*pg.119*
28	Carrot Baked Oatmeal	Black Bean Risotto	Tilapia with Tomatoes and Pepper Relish	Salad of Kale, Avocado, and Carrots
	pg.19	*pg.45*	*pg.84*	*pg.114*
29	Spinach & Egg Scramble with Raspberries	Grilled Chicken Breasts with Plum Salsa	Shrimp and Rice Noodle Salad	Quinoa Spinach Power Salad
	pg.19	*pg.59*	*pg.108*	*pg.113*
30	Egg Tartine	Oven Roasted Salmon Fillets	Creamy Quinoa, Lentils and Vegetables	Wilted Spinach and Tilapia Salad
30	*pg.27*	*pg.56*	*pg.106*	*pg.121*

Your Foodlist

Thank you for embarking on a journey to a healthier heart with our "**Heart Healthy Cookbook for Beginners**." To enhance your experience and make your transition to heart-healthy eating as seamless as possible, we are delighted to present an exclusive bonus just for you.

How to Access Your Bonus

1. **Scan the QR Code** with your smartphone's camera to access.

2. **Download your** personalized **Heart-Healthy Grocery Foodlist**.

This carefully curated list complements the recipes in our cookbook, ensuring you have all the nutritious ingredients you need.

Made in United States
Troutdale, OR
01/06/2024